ULTRASOUND OF THE CHEST

A guide for clinicians

Ultrasound of the Chest

A guide for clinicians

William Kinnear and
Maruti Kumaran

Queens Medical Centre, Nottingham

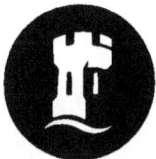

Nottingham
University Press

First published by Nottingham University Press
This reissued original edition published 2023 by 5m Books Ltd www.5mbooks.com

British Library Cataloguing in Publication Data
Ultrasound of the Chest - A guide for clinicians
I. Kinnear, William J.M; II. Kumaran, M.

ISBN 9781789183207

Disclaimer

Every reasonable effort has been made to ensure that the material in this book is true, correct, complete
and appropriate at the time of writing. Nevertheless the publishers and the author do not accept
responsibility for any omission or error, or for any injury, damage, loss or financial consequences arising
from the use of the book. Views expressed in the articles are those of the author and not of the Editor or
Publisher.

Typeset by Nottingham University Press, Nottingham

EU GPSR Authorised Representative
LOGOS EUROPE, 9 rue Nicolas Poussin, 17000, LA ROCHELLE, France
E-mail: Contact@logoseurope.eu

Contents

Introduction

Portable ultrasound devices will be in use in many different places around your hospital – for scanning bladders, inserting central venous lines, assessing trauma patients etc. Bedside ultrasound scanning is changing our approach to respiratory patients, particularly those with pleural disease.

This is a guide for clinicians, to help you learn how to ultrasound the chest. Later on we will look at some more advanced applications to give you an idea of what a skilled radiologist with a more powerful instrument can do, but mostly we will stick with a simple scanner at the bedside.

This book is about trans-thoracic ultrasound. We will not cover endo-bronchial techniques.

1
Basics

What is ultrasound?

Sound waves are vibrations of particulate matter, which produce alternate areas of compression and rarefaction. They need a medium in which to travel and cannot pass through a vacuum.

Sound waves are sometimes depicted as sine waves, with the parameters of amplitude and wavelength.

How are ultrasound waves produced?

The core of ultrasound is the piezo-electric crystal. The crystal, or array of crystals, converts a pulse of electricity into a pulse of ultrasound. These are the same crystals that run in quartz watches.

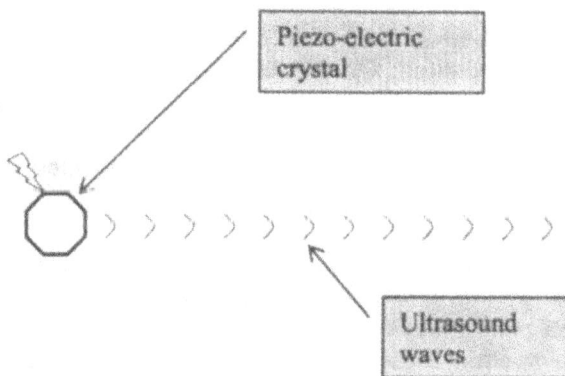

Piezo-electric crystal

Ultrasound waves

Figure 1.1 Ultrasound waves produced by applying a pulse of electricity to a piezo-electric crystal.

Frequency and wavelength

The human ear can hear sound waves of a frequency between about 20 and 20,000 cycles per second (a cycle per second is called Hertz, or Hz for short). "Ultra"sound refers to waves of frequency higher than 20,000 Hz, beyond the human acoustic range. In clinical practice, ultrasound frequencies are measured in Mega-Hertz (MHz), one MHz being 1,000,000 Hz.

Higher frequencies give pictures of higher resolution, but do not penetrate very far into tissues. Lower frequencies penetrate better but give poorer resolution. The probes used for superficial ultrasound – for example to guide intravenous line placement – use higher frequencies than those we usually use for scanning the chest.

Acoustic impedance

Sound waves have a constant speed in any homogenous medium, but this varies between media depending on the density and elasticity of the matter in the medium.

The velocity of sound in water and soft tissues is very similar at about 1500 meters/second. Sound travels more slowly in air – around 500 meters/second.

The way in which sound passes through a medium is called its "acoustic impedance". This depends on how dense the medium is and how fast sounds travels in it.

Bone and air are poor conductors of ultrasound.

Acoustic reflection

Sound waves tend to be reflected when there is an interface of two media of different acoustic impedances. The greater the difference in acoustic impedance, the more sound waves are reflected. Water and soft tissues have very similar acoustic impedances, whereas the impedance of air – or bone - is very different, so the ultrasound waves are reflected back. These reflected waves are called echoes.

In a moment we will look at a patient with a pleural effusion. The ultrasound waves pass through the ultrasound gel on the surface of the chest, the soft tissues (which are mainly made up of water) and the pleural fluid; all these have similar acoustic impedances, so very little of the ultrasound is reflected. When the ultrasound hits the air-filled lung, the acoustic impedance is very different, which causes the waves to be reflected back out towards the probe.

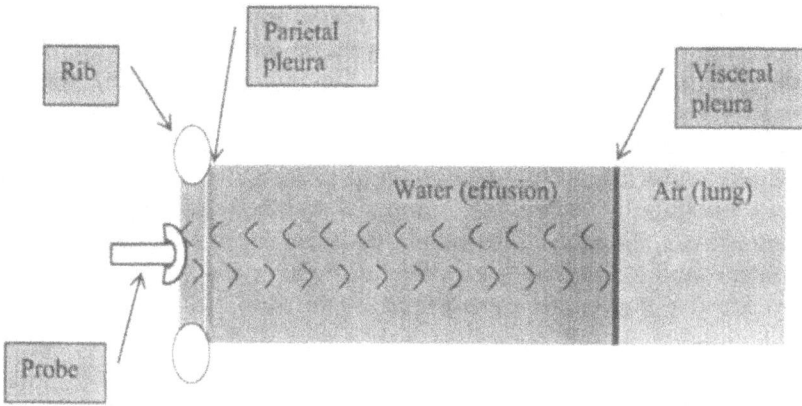

Figure 1.2 Reflection of ultrasound waves at the interface between media with different sound-conducting properties.

Measuring Distance

When the reflected ultrasound gets back to the piezo-electric crystal again, it vibrates it and induces a small electric current. After some sophisticated processing, this signal provides the basis of the picture we see on our screen.

The time it takes for the ultrasound waves to travel to the reflector and back is used to work out how far away the reflector is: the further away, the more time it will take. This is similar to the echo you hear when a loud noise, such as a hand-clap, bounces back to your ears from a wall some distance away; if you are out in the countryside, there is usually no hard reflective surface, so you don't hear an echo when you clap. (You don't hear an echo when you are in a small room, because the time delay is too short for our brains to detect.)

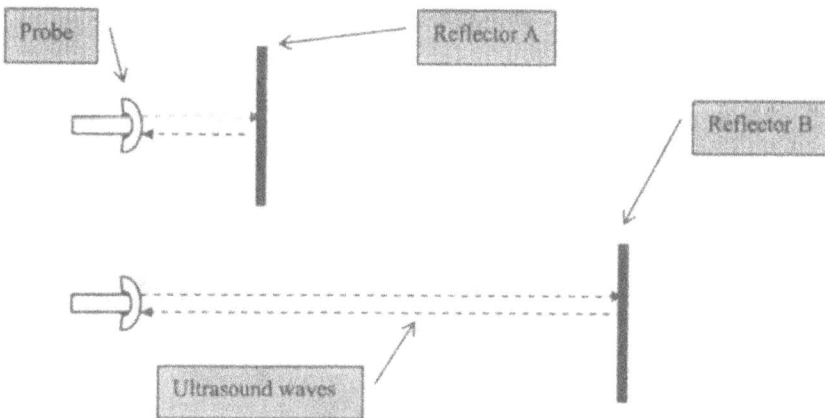

Figure 1.3 Measuring distance using echoes. Sound waves reflected by an interface further away take longer to get back to the probe.

One last bit about the generation of the sound waves. If you produce sound waves by striking a large bell, the sound goes on for a few seconds. The piezo-electric crystal acts both as the source of the sound, and as the microphone listening for returning echoes. Whilst our bell (or piezo-electric crystal) is resonating, it cannot "hear" the vibrations produced by reflected echoes. In order to overcome this problem, we have to dampen the vibrations so that they die down very quickly. With a bell you could do this by putting a cloth inside it: when you strike it the pitch of the note is the same, but it dies away very quickly. In an ultrasound probe, the piezo-electric crystals are backed by absorbent material which achieves the same effect.

The whole picture

So, let's summarise the physics so far:

- A pulse of electricity is passed across the piezo-electric crystal in the probe, which causes it to produce a brief pulse of very high frequency sound waves.
- These waves shoot off into the tissues.
- The piezo-electric crystal waits and listens for any echoes.
- If the ultrasound waves hit an interface between two tissues with different acoustic impedances (sound-conducting properties), they are reflected back towards the probe.
- When any reflected ultrasound waves hit the piezo-electric crystal again, they produce an electric current.
- The time delay before the reflected echoes return tells us how far away the reflective surface was.
- Another pulse of ultrasound is produced, to obtain the next frame of the image.

In our picture of ultrasound waves emitted from a probe, it would be more accurate to depict the sound waves grouped in pulses.

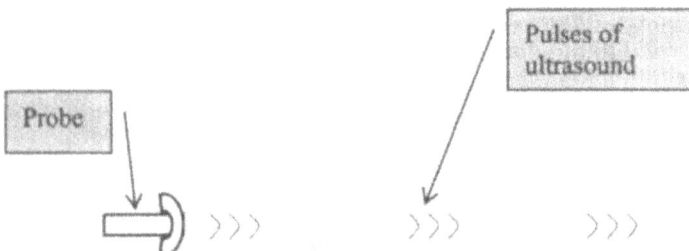

Figure 1.4 Pulses of ultrasound produced by the piezo-electric crystals in an ultrasound probe. Between pulses, the probe "listens" for returning echoes.

If you now imagine a whole line of piezo-electric crystals in a row – an array – you can see how we could create a single snap-shot picture of the tissues underneath our probe. The abdominal probe we will use for most chest imaging is a curved array, whereas the smaller vascular probes are linear arrays. It only takes a fraction of a second to take this picture, so we can take lots of them in quick succession to make a movie: real-time ultrasound. For the record, this is called B Mode – let's not worry about A and M mode scans for the moment.

Black and White

Figure 1.5 is the sort of image you might see when you first ultrasound the chest.

This patient has a pleural effusion. The bright white line is the visceral pleural, where there is a reflective interface, because the lung (air) and the pleural effusion (water) have very different acoustic impedances

On a plain CXR, water blocks the transmission of X-rays, so a pleural effusion appears white (whereas a pneumothorax is black because the rays pass through unimpeded). Ultrasound waves are transmitted by water so a pleural effusion will appear black on your screen.

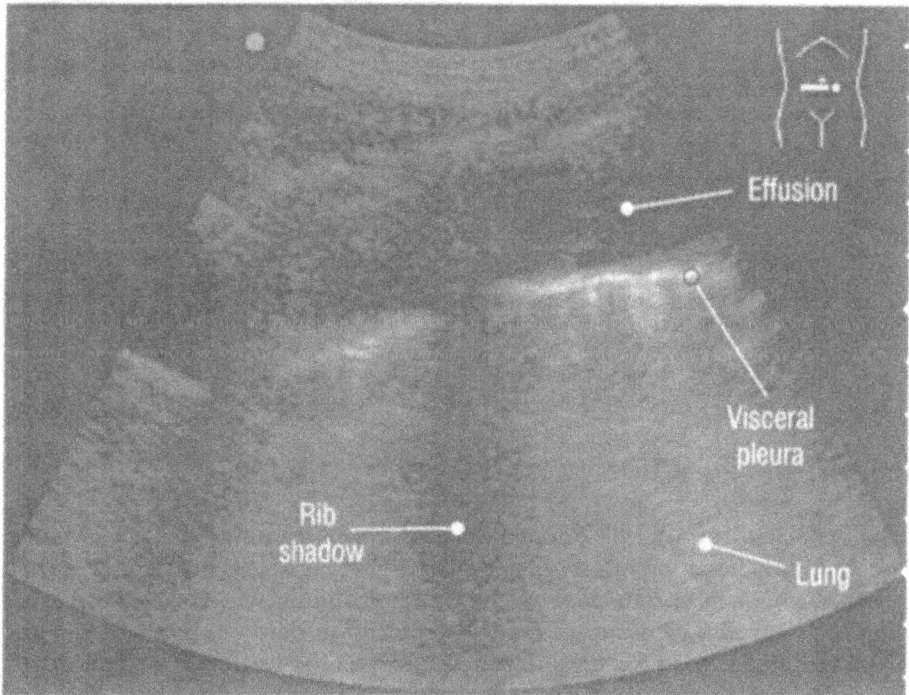

Figure 1.5 Acoustic reflection from the interface between pleural fluid and lung. The interface appears bright, whereas the pleural fluid – which conducts rather than reflects ultrasound – is black.

Acoustic shadows

If most of the ultrasound beam is reflected by an object, there will be an acoustic "shadow" behind the object. You will see this fairly early on with rib shadows, where the difference in acoustic impedance between bone and the surrounding soft tissues causes the ultrasound waves to be reflected rather than transmitted.

The structures that normally cause shadowing are air, bones or structures with calcium deposition – all with very different acoustic impedances to water (and soft tissues, which we have already noted consist mainly of water).

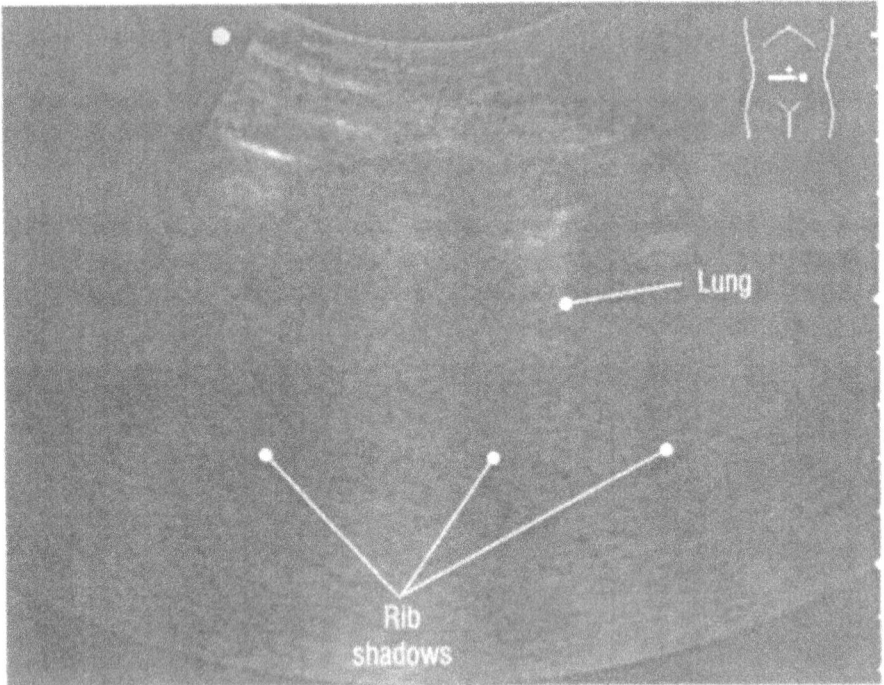

Figure 1.6 Acoustic shadows behind ribs. The ultrasound waves are not conducted by bone, so there is a dark area behind each rib.

Scatter: Black, White .... and Grey

A flat reflective surface will bounce most of the ultrasound back towards the probe. If the ultrasound hits a reflector that is smaller or less flat, the waves are scattered rather than reflected. Some of the scattered waves will travel back towards the probe, whereas others will shoot off in different directions. They will all be smaller than the original wave which hit the tissue. The small waves which get back to the probe are represented as smaller reflections – they are less bright than those from a strong reflector, and appear grey rather than white. This is why the lungs, liver etc appear grey.

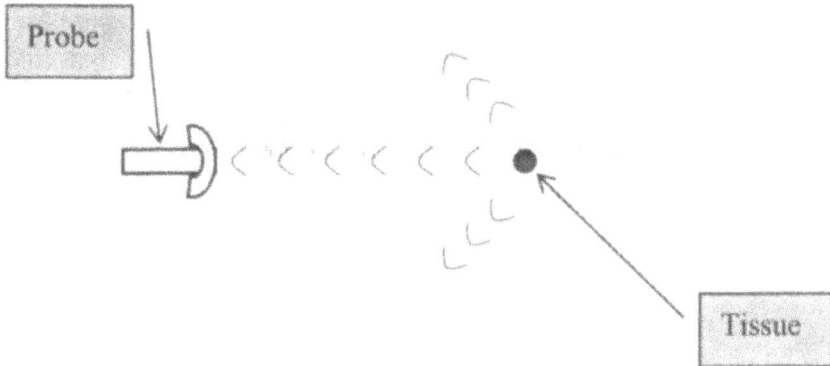

Figure 1.7 Scatter of ultrasound in tissue. Some of the scattered ultrasound returns back to the probe, resulting in some brightness – but not as much as if all the ultrasound had been reflected back.

Artefacts

Some of the things we see on ultrasound are real anatomical structures, like the pleural space. Artefacts are misrepresentation of echoes in relation to the actual structures. Examples are reverberation, comet-tail and mirror artefacts. We'll talk about these in more detail later on.

Bio-effects

When ripples spread out over the surface of a pond, they gradually become smaller and eventually disappear. The same thing happens to ultrasound waves in tissue, a process which is called attenuation. The energy of the sound waves is changed into heat in the tissues, so there is a theoretical possibility of tissue damage. In practice, this effect on tissue is so small that it can be ignored. Diagnostic ultrasound is perfectly safe.

2
Settings

Before we scan our first patient, let's look at some of the settings on the machine. A good way to explore these is to scan yourself, and one of the easiest things to see is your liver. (The pleura is much more difficult to see, unless you have a pleural effusion.) You can do this holding the probe in one hand, leaving the other free to adjust the settings on the machine.

So, select an abdominal probe (if you have the choice), switch the scanner on, apply lots of gel to the probe and put it over your right lower rib-cage anteriorly, with the probe aligned vertically. Slide the probe up and down until you find your liver.

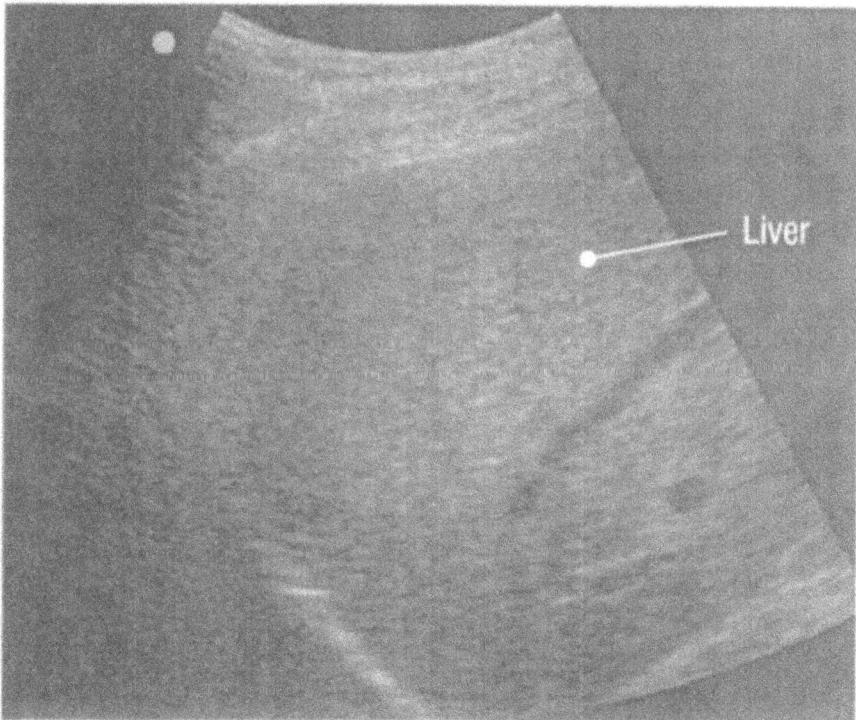

Figure 2.1 Normal liver.

Depth

Your scanner may allow you to adjust the depth of the scan. If you adjust this sequentially, you will see how your liver is progressively magnified.

At the most shallow setting, take some deep breaths in and out and see if you can observe the liver sliding along the ribs.

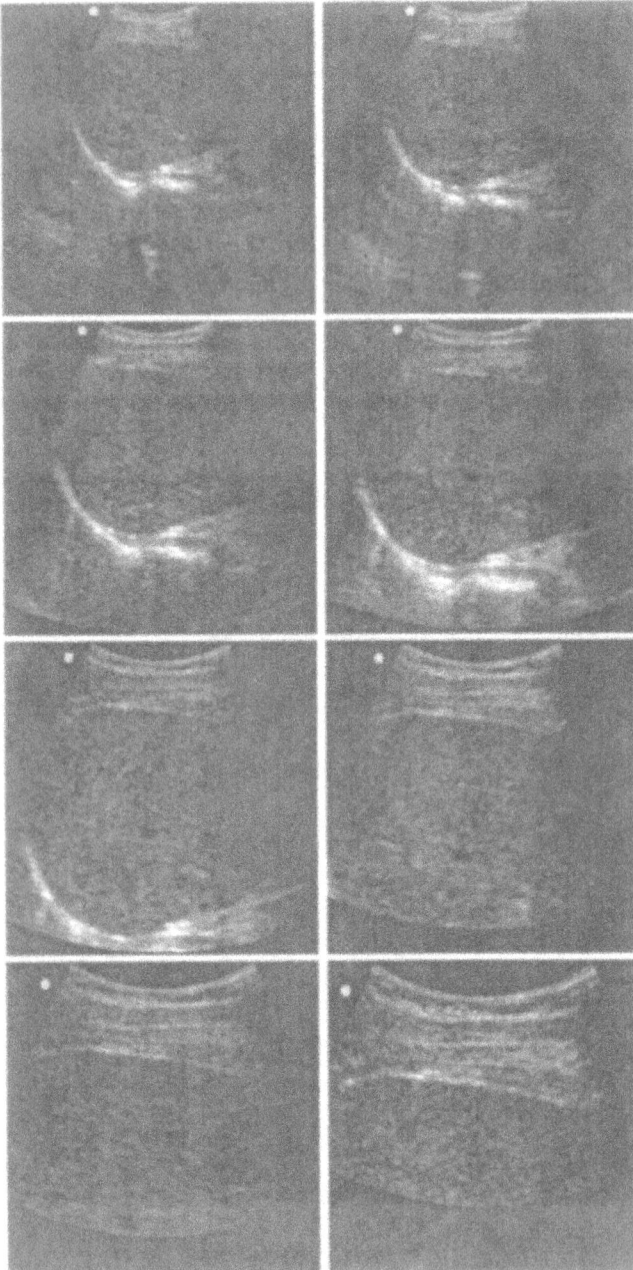

Figure 2.2 Effect of adjusting the depth settings. The intercostal space is progressively magnified, and the deeper structures lost.

Gain

You can turn up the gain on the screen of your ultrasound machine, in just the same way you can adjust the brightness of the image on any digital device. There may be an "auto-gain" facility, to help you optimise the picture, but you may need to make your own gain adjustments from time to time. How you adjust the gain will depend on what you are looking at. There are no hard-and-fast rules about gain – if you turn it up and down during your first few scans, you will see how this adjustment changes the definition of the picture. You want the grey bits to be grey, not completely black or white. Some scanners allow you to change the gain of the deeper and shallower parts of the image independently.

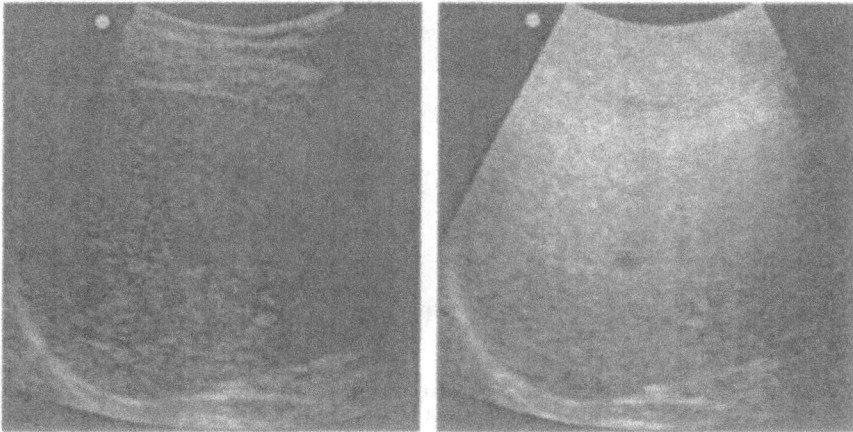

Figure 2.3 Effect of gain on definition.
The left image is too dark, the right one too bright.

Focus

You may be able to select the region of focus on your scanner. This allows you to see the area you are interested in with better definition.

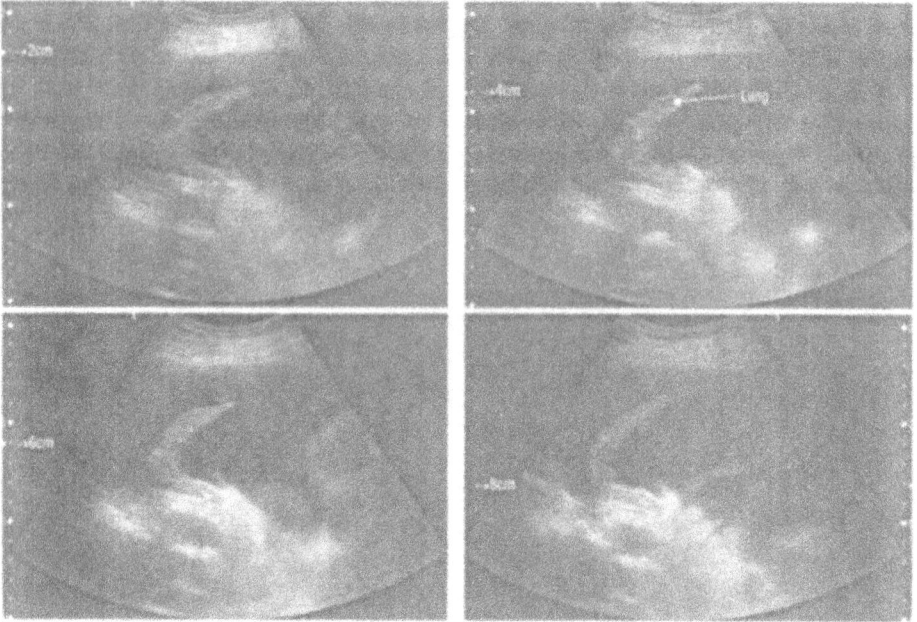

Figure 2.4 Effect of adjusting the depth of focus on definition. On this scan, the lung is seen less clearly when the focal depth – indicated by the arrow on the left of the scan – is too deep (bottom right) or too shallow (top left).

Penetration

With abdominal probes, there may be a choice of penetration. In a very obese subject, you may get better images if you choose the "Penetrated" setting: the scanner switches to a lower frequency of ultrasound which aids penetration (at the cost of resolution). Conversely in "Resolution" mode, a higher frequency will give better resolution but poorer penetration into deeper structures.

Measurement

When you have a clear image of your liver, freeze the screen, turn the measurement cursor on and measure the diameter of your liver.

There will be lots of other facilities, for example allowing you to write text on the image, save images etc, but let's stick to the basics for the moment.

You could scan a few different people, until you are conversant with the controls on your scanner, but a lot of the things we have been discussing will make more sense when you start to scan patients with pleural effusions.

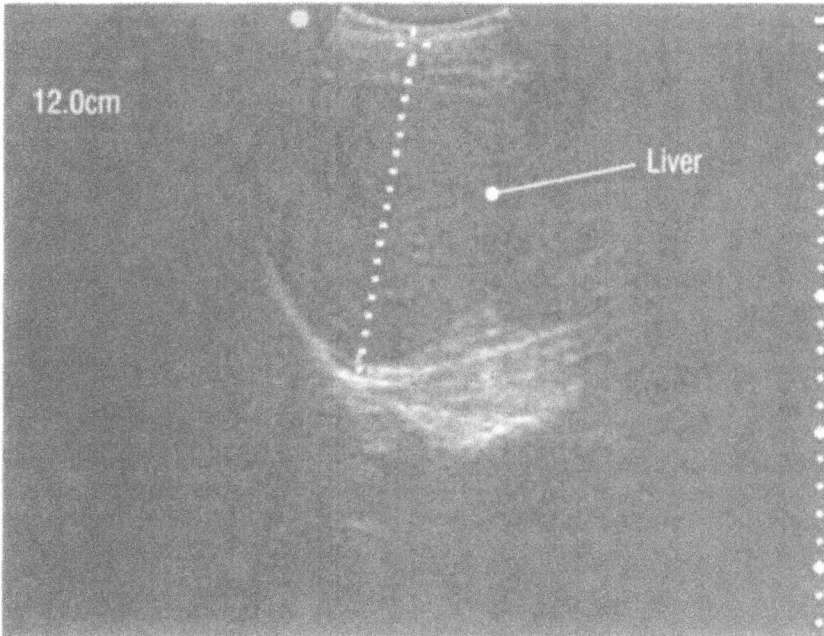

Figure 2.5 Measuring distance on an ultrasound scan.

3

Pleural Effusions

For your first scan, choose a patient with a chest X-ray or CT scan which shows a large pleural effusion.

Hygiene

It is possible to perform ultrasound under sterile conditions, for example when guiding a biopsy needle, but most of the time it is a "clean" rather than sterile procedure. We'll talk about ultrasound-guided biopsy later.

Before you perform an ultrasound examination, wash your hands thoroughly. Clean the probe using alcohol hand-cleansing gel on a clean paper towel. At the end of the examination, wipe the ultrasound gel (see next section) off the probe using paper towels and then clean it using alcohol gel.

Gel

Ultrasound gel has the same acoustic impedance as soft tissues. It "couples" the probe to the patient, conducting the ultrasound waves from the transducer into the tissues. Other sorts of gel might look the same – lubricants, hand-cleansing solutions, etc - but they don't work. Use lots of gel, but remember to wipe it off the patient afterwards.

- Position the patient – sitting up, or lying on their side with the effusion uppermost.
- Wash your hands.
- Turn on your ultrasound machine.
- If you have a choice of probes, use the one designed for abdominal scanning.
- Clean the probe.
- Apply lots of ultrasound gel to the patient's chest.
- Put the probe on the patient. A good place to start is around the anterior axillary line, at right-angles to the ribs (ie with the probe vertical if the patient is sitting, horizontal if they are lying down).

- Adjust the gain so that the picture looks neither too black nor too white.

- Slide the probe up and down the rib-cage, to orientate yourself as to which direction is which on the screen.

Rib shadows

The first thing you will notice is that there are some black bands across the screen which fan out from the probe. These move as you slide the probe up and down. They are shadows caused by the ribs, which block the ultrasound waves, as we saw in the last chapter. For the moment, concentrate on what you see between these shadows.

Pleural fluid

Pleural fluid doesn't reflect ultrasound, and so a simple pleural effusion will appear as a black area.

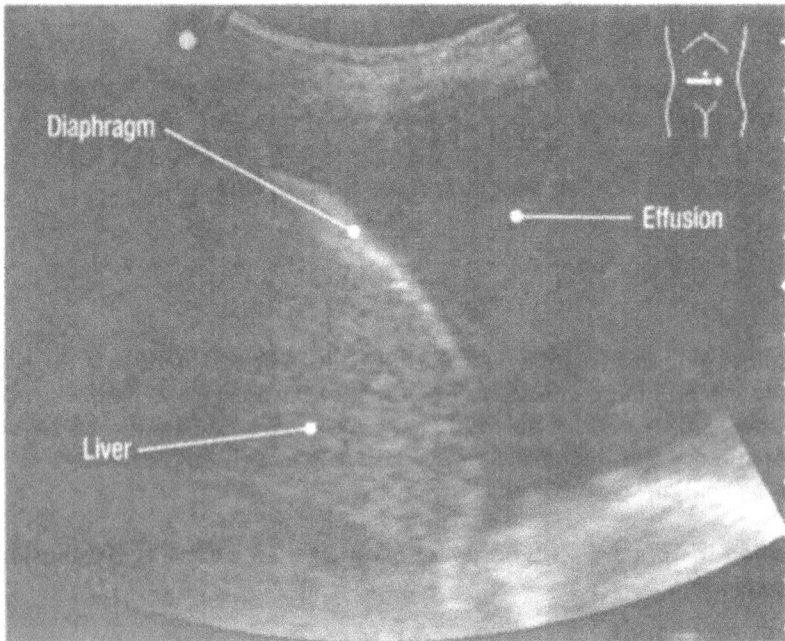

Figure 3.1 A large right pleural effusion, indicated by the black area above the liver.

Liver and Spleen

Over the right hemi-thorax, if you slide the probe down towards the abdomen, you should encounter a liver. This is grey, with ducts and vessels within it, as we have seen already. If you are on the left side of the chest, you may see the spleen; it is situated posteriorly, and is more difficult to see than the liver.

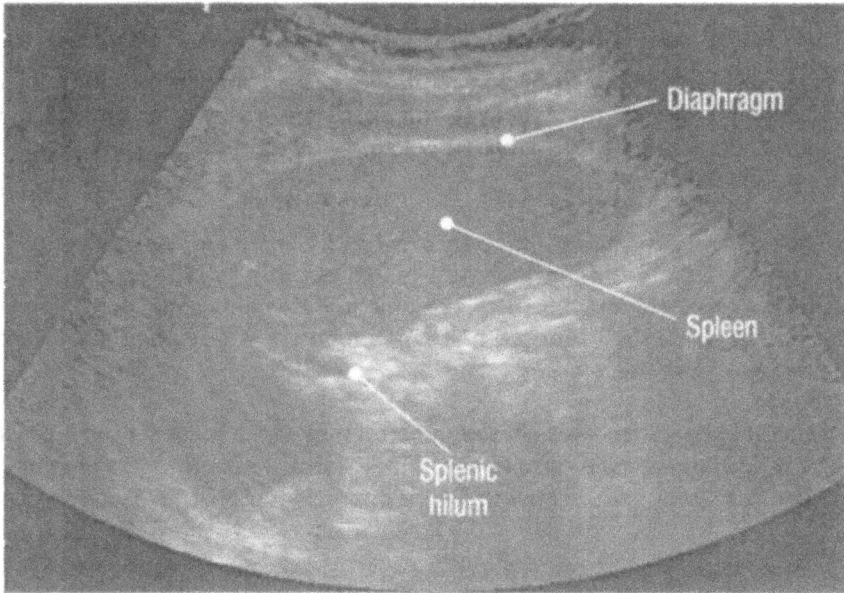

Figure 3.2 The spleen below a left pleural effusion.

Diaphragm

One crucial appearance to note is that of the diaphragm - two white lines separated by a black line.

Being able to identify the diaphragm is essential when it comes to pleural aspiration, insertion of a chest drain or thoracoscopy.

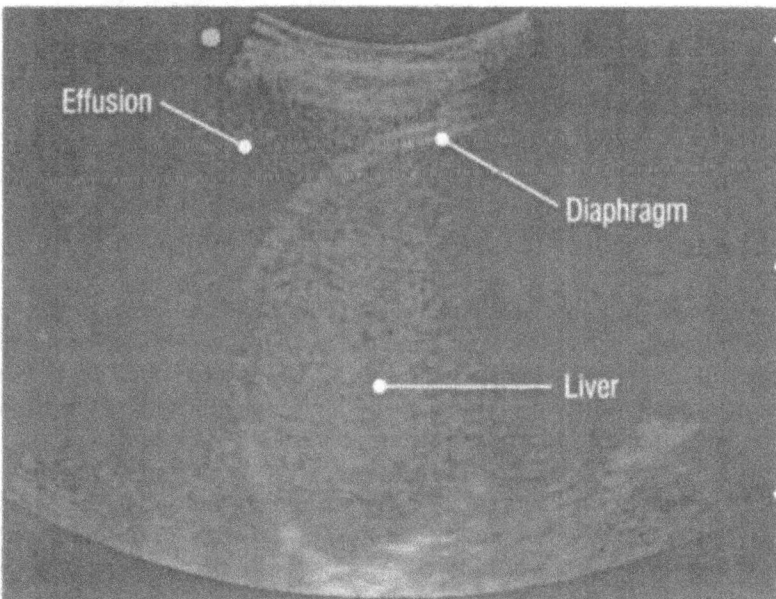

Figure 3.3 The diaphragm – a black line sandwiched by two white lines.

Pleural effusions

So, we have learnt to look between rib shadows; we can identify a large pleural effusion, with diaphragm and liver/spleen below it. Let's look at a smaller effusion. Just like the large effusion we started with, this is a dark, echo-free area on the scan.

You should now be getting the idea of what pleural fluid looks like. As you gain experience in scanning the chest, you'll be able to pick up even smaller effusions. With experience, you will be able to detect tiny collections – perhaps a few tens of millilitres – that are not visible on a chest X-ray and are too small to be detected clinically.

It is difficult to judge from an ultrasound scan how much pleural fluid is present. There are formulae which use the two-dimensional measurements of your scan to estimate a volume, but they are very imprecise and of little use in clinical practice.

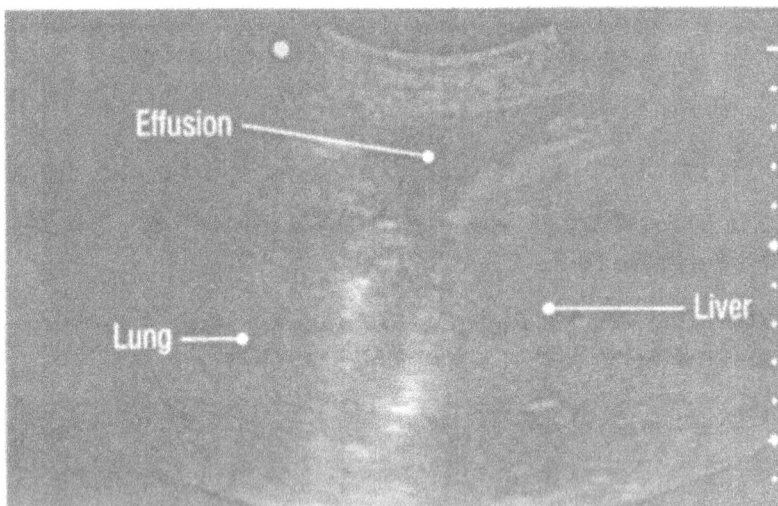

Figure 3.4 A small pleural effusion.

Pleural aspiration

Taking into account the clinical picture, you can decide whether or not to do a diagnostic tap on an effusion, even if it is quite small. Moving the probe around will show you the best site to aspirate, where there is most fluid. Try to keep the probe exactly perpendicular to the skin when you select your site for aspiration: this is the easiest line to reproduce when you insert your needle.

You can use the distance markers on the scanner to guide you as to how far you will need to put your needle in, and how far it is safe to go before you run the risk of hitting the visceral pleura. Mark the site on the skin, wipe off the ultrasound gel from the patient and clean the probe. Then perform pleural aspiration exactly as you would normally.

Ultrasound at the bedside works much better than the "X marks the spot" technique, where the scan in done in the imaging department but the patient is then transferred back up to ward for the aspiration to be performed. It is difficult to be sure that the patient is in exactly the same position and that the probe is in the same orientation as your aspiration needle.

This is not a textbook on pleural fluid, but just a reminder of the six basic things to send pleural fluid for:

- Microscopy and culture
- Cytology
- pH
- Protein
- LDH
- Glucose

Of course, if you aspirate frank pus then only the first of these is important.

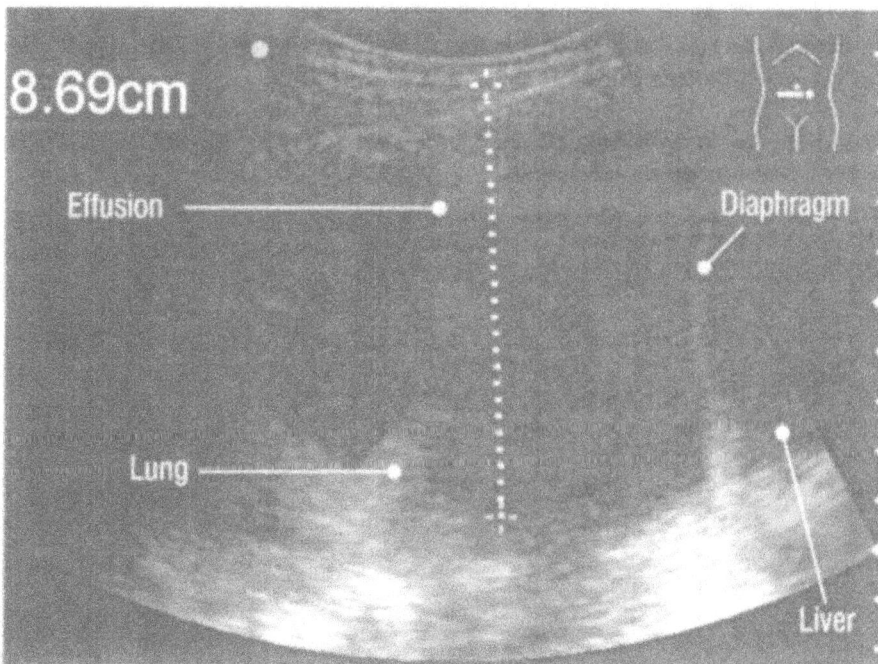

Figure 3.5 Measuring the depth of a pleural effusion.

The intercostal artery, as you will doubtless remember, runs underneath the rib in the sub-costal groove. It is important to realise that it only gets into the groove around the posterior axillary line; more posterior to this point, it is in the middle of the intercostal space. You should try and avoid aspiration sites that are further round towards the back than the posterior axillary line.

If you have the facility to detect flow using Doppler on your scanner, you can check to see where the intercostal artery is before you perform the procedure. Vascular Doppler usually utilises the colours blue and red to differentiate the direction of flow. When we are scanning the chest, the direction of flow is not usually important, so use the Power Doppler setting which is more sensitive to flow.

Doppler can also be used to differentiate pleural thickening from a pleural effusion: you may be able to see the exudate fluid swilling around with respiration on a Doppler scan.

Complicated effusions and empyema

Once you start ultrasounding the chest, you will soon find yourself looking at difficult effusions, for example after a failed attempt at aspiration. These are much harder than the large uncomplicated effusion that you chose for your first case.

Sometimes you will be able to show that there is no pleural fluid – it is not uncommon to find that the clinical impression of pleural effusion was wrong. For example, if the right hemi-diaphragm is elevated then with ultrasound you may be able to see the liver at the site of dullness to percussion. (We'll move onto the appearances of pneumonia in a little while.)

Rather than being uniformly black, the pleural fluid may appear grey, because it is thick and therefore echogenic.

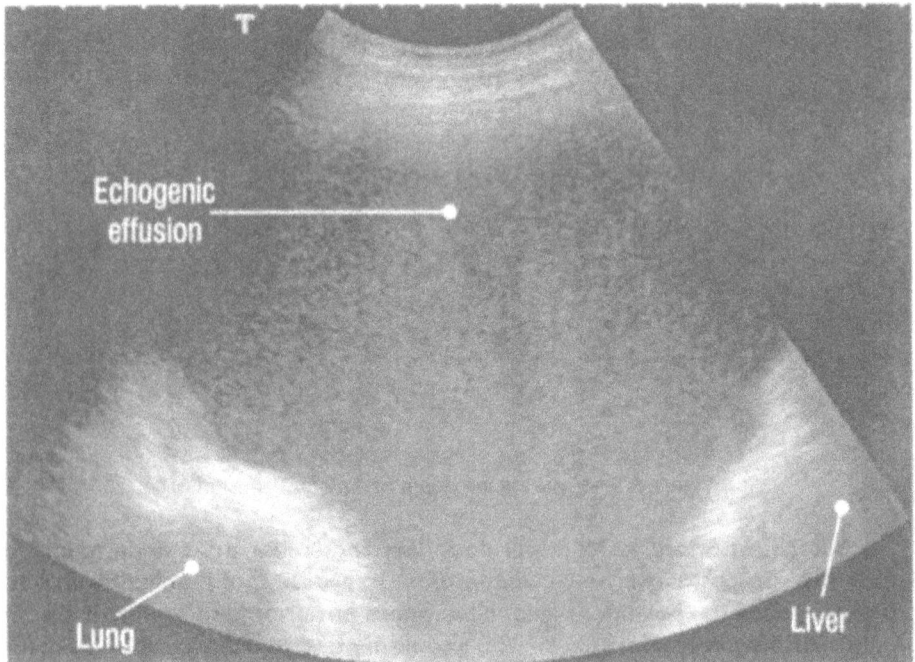

Figure 3.6 Echogenic pleural fluid.

White specks within the fluid indicate the presence of air, showing that the effusion is likely to be an empyema caused by anerobic gas-forming bacteria – or that a small amount of air has got in during a previous aspiration.

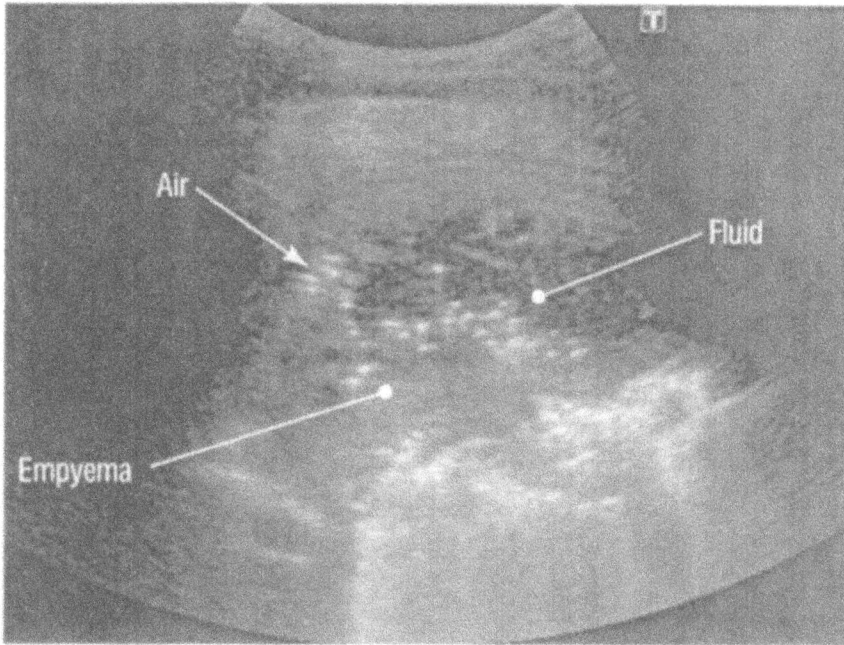

Figure 3.7 Air within an empyema.

Pleural thickening tells you that the effusion is likely to be an exudate. We'll return to look at the pleura in more detail later.

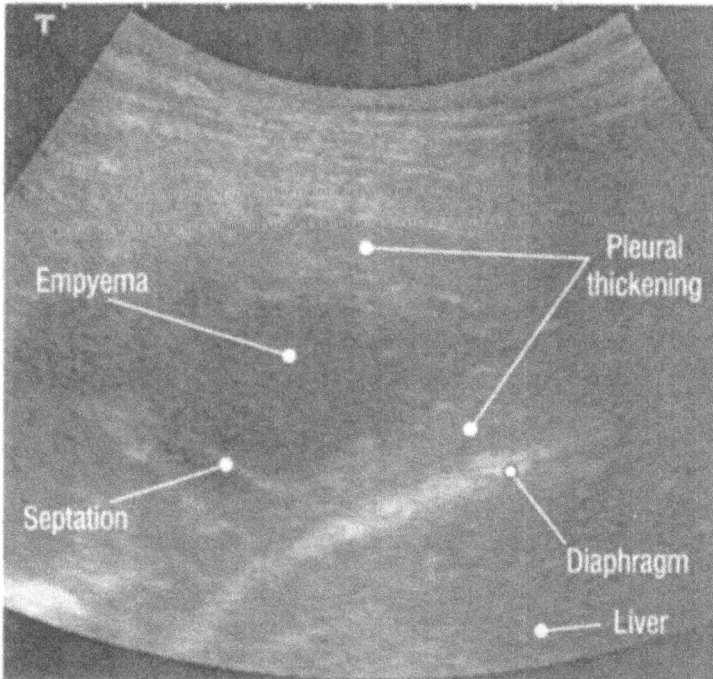

Figure 3.8 An exudative pleural effusion with pleural thickening.

Loculated effusions will have white bands running across the dark areas of fluid. These do not necessarily mean that the pleural effusion is an empyema – it is quite common to see thin bands in an uncomplicated para-pneumonic effusion.

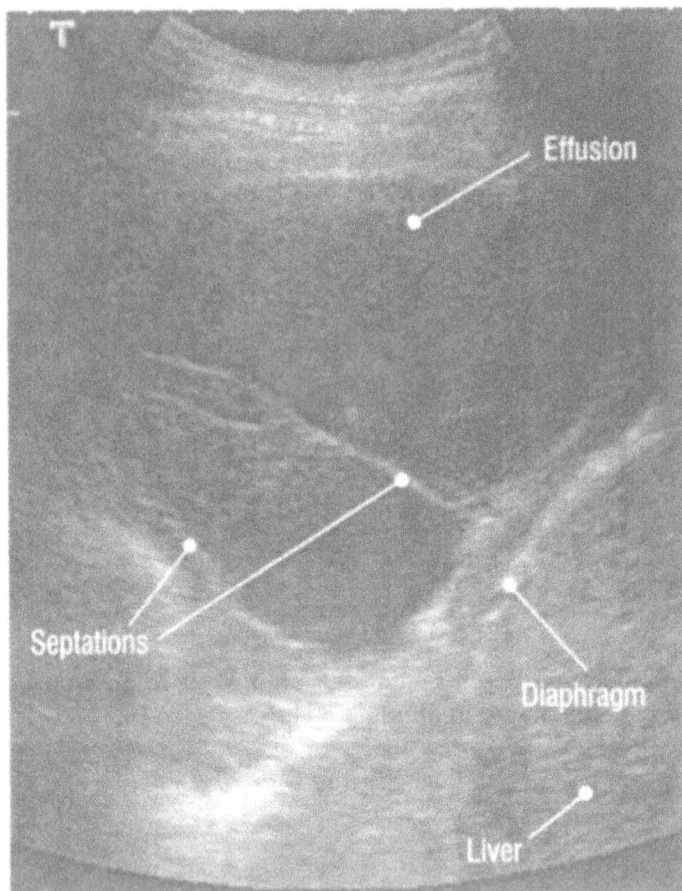

Figure 3.9 Loculations within a pleural effusion. The white lines are fibrinous septations.

Sometimes the whole effusion may appear quite solid. Ultrasound can show you where to aspirate if you need a diagnostic sample of pleural fluid, but a CT scan may be more help in deciding about drainage or surgery.

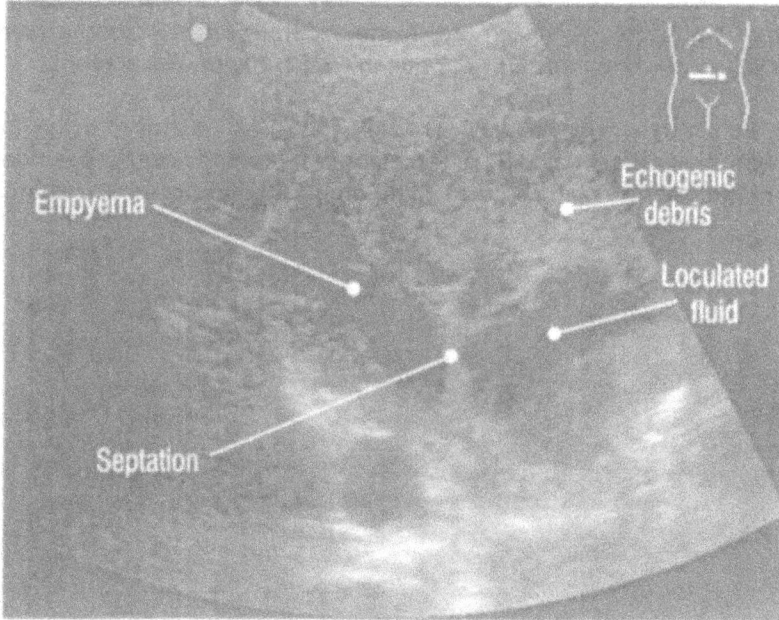

Figure 3.10 Complex empyema. The dark areas are pockets of fluid, separated by thick septations and more solid areas.

The Next Level

If you are just starting to ultrasound the chest, this would be a good point to pause until you feel you can confidently identify a pleural effusion. You will need someone to supervise you for your first ten or so scans. Then do at least another ten by yourself. You should be able to find the liver/spleen and diaphragm reliably every time, to see a pleural effusion if there is one present or to be confident that there is no fluid there.

You may, quite reasonably, decide that this is the level of competency you wish to achieve. After all, the main role of bedside chest ultrasound is to identify the best site for diagnostic aspiration or insertion of a chest drain (or thoracoscope). If you read on, you will find out about other things you may see when scanning the chest, anatomical appearances or artefacts. It would do no harm to be aware of them, even if you are going to limit your practice to looking for pleural fluid.

In the next section we'll look at pneumonia: as we've already discussed, one reason you may be asked to ultrasound the chest is because someone has looked at a CXR and thought there was a pleural effusion, but failed to obtain any fluid when attempting a diagnostic aspiration – a "dry tap". This could be because the site chosen according to physical signs was wrong, but the cause of the CXR shadowing might be pneumonia rather than effusion. As you become better at ultrasound, you may be able to recognise the appearances of pneumonia and make a positive diagnosis, rather than just excluding pleural fluid.

After that we'll look at the pleura in more detail, and talk about comet-tail artefacts (those white lines that appear so frequently on you screen).

Finally, we'll move on to the ribs and lymph nodes. As we stray into the preserve of skilled radiologists, we end by reflecting on what can and cannot be undertaken safely at the bedside by a clinician using a portable ultrasound machine.

4

Pneumonia

When you have scanned pleural effusions, you may have seen the characteristic white triangular shape of compressed lung.

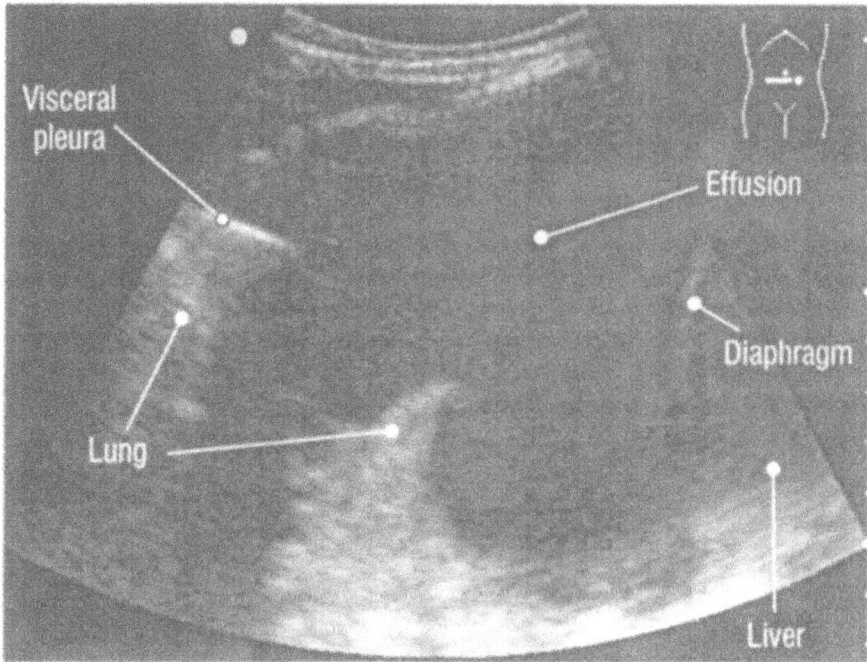

Figure 4.1 Atelectasis. The lung appears as a white object within the black pleural fluid.

Consolidated lung (Figure 4.2) has white specks within it. These white specks are air-filled bronchi, surrounded by solid lung: on a chest X-ray this would be an air-bronchogram. The interface between the air and the consolidated lung is highly reflective, hence the white specks.

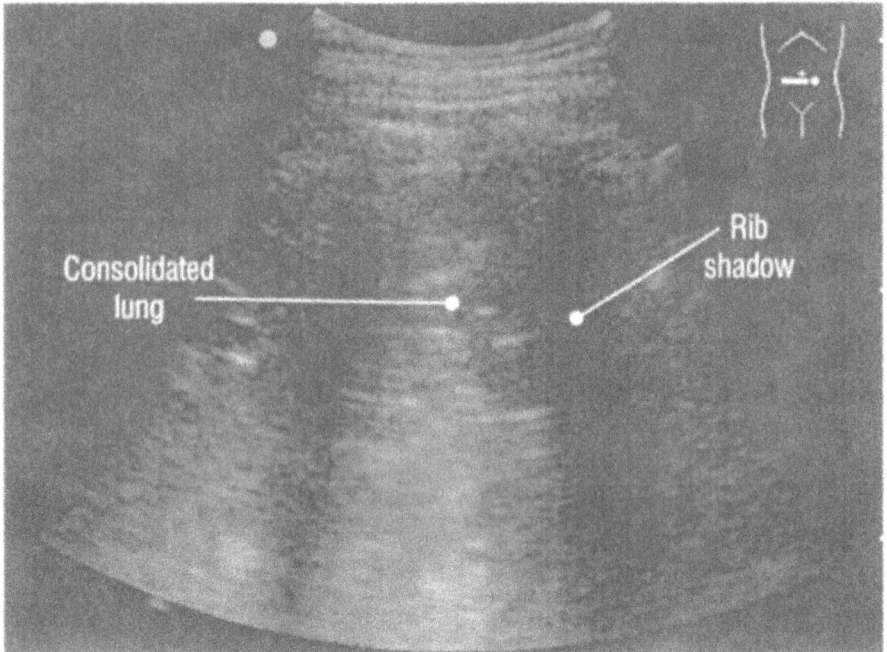

Figure 4.2 Pneumonia.

When we started looking at pleural effusions, we noticed how ultrasound was reflected at the visceral pleura where there was an interface between two tissues with different sound-conducting properties – pleural effusion (water) and lung (air). The white areas in consolidation have the same explanation: ultrasound that is reflected at the interface between air (in the bronchi) and solid tissue (consolidated lung). You don't see bronchi normally because they contain air and are surrounded by air (in the lung), so there is no reflective interface.

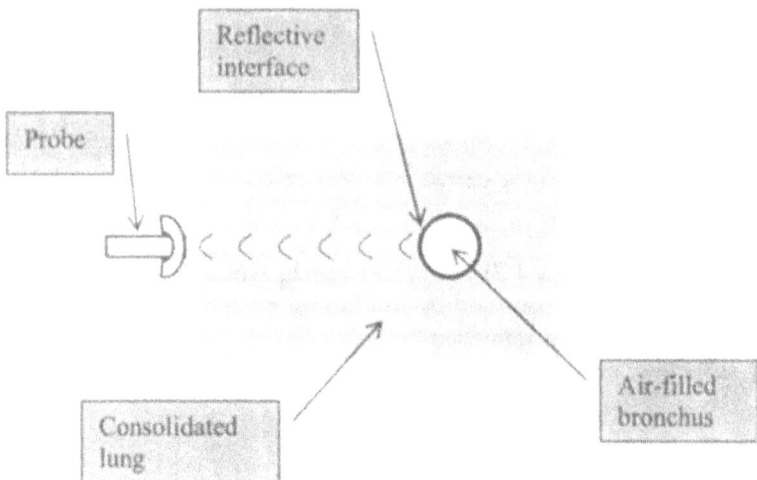

Figure 4.3 Reflection of ultrasound by bronchial air in consolidated lung.

If you catch a bronchus longitudinally, you will see a longer white tube.

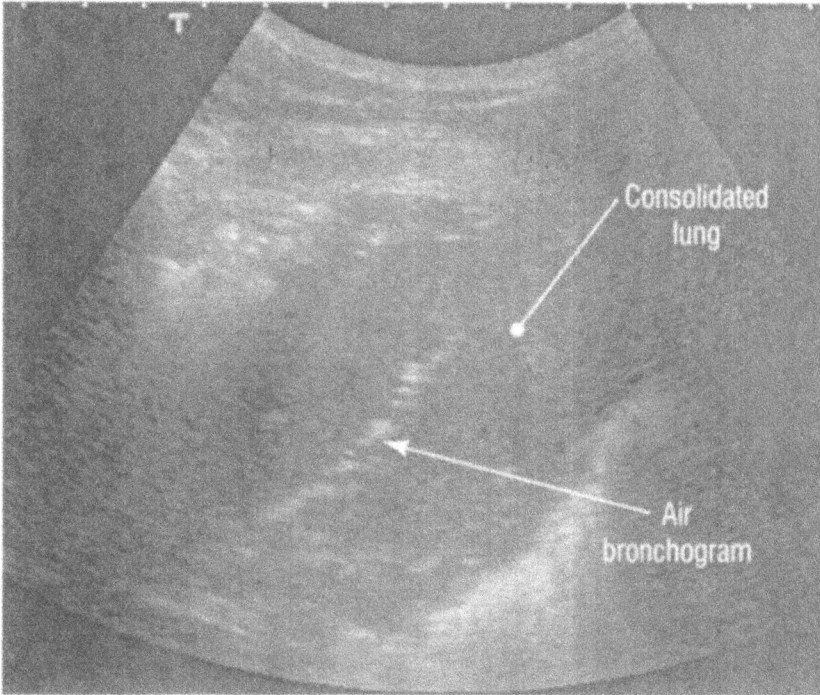

Figure 4.4 Air-bronchogram.

If the bronchus is full of pus, then it will be black rather than white. You may be able to see large fluid-filled bronchi if there is bronchiectasis.

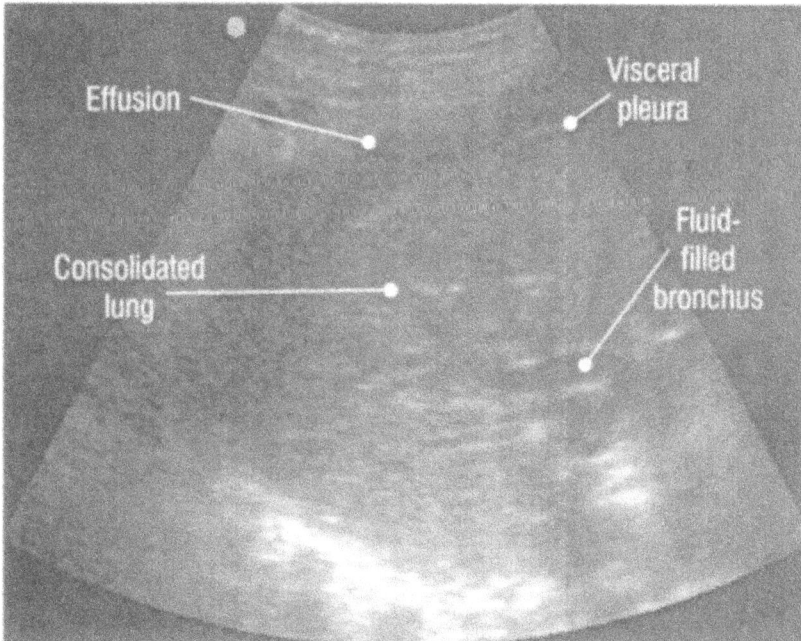

Figure 4.5 Fluid-filled bronchus.

5

Heart Failure

Heart failure is a common cause of a pleural effusion. If you see fluid in the pleural space on both sides of the chest, heart failure becomes much more likely.

There is nothing particularly characteristic about the appearance of the fluid on ultrasound, but if the underlying lung is oedematous you may see a lot of white lines spreading out from the visceral pleura to the edge of your screen. These are called comet-tail artefacts.

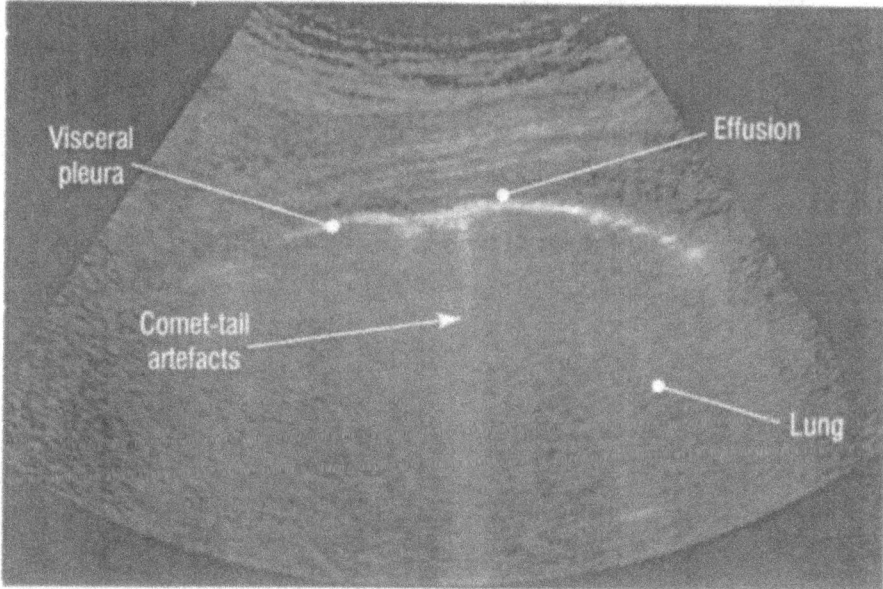

Figure 5.1 Comet-tail artefacts in heart failure. These white lines arise at the pleural surface and radiate out to the edge of the screen.

Comet-tails

"Comet-tail" artefacts are white lines which run from the pleura down to the edge of your screen (Figure 5.1). Comets are pretty uncommon – maybe the vapour trail of a jet aeroplane in the sky would be a more useful analogy.

Comet-tail artefacts are less well understood than other artefacts, although one suggestion is that they represent reverberation between interlobular septa. We'll discuss reverberation in more detail in chapter 8.

There may be several comet-tails. As a general rule, more than six in any one screen indicates pathology. In the presence of a pneumothorax, comet-tail artefacts disappear.

Comet-tail artefacts are also numerous in other conditions such as tuberculosis, sarcoidosis or other diseases which cause pleural irregularity. You'll see them on quite a few of the scans in this book.

Pericardial fluid

If you want to look at the heart using ultrasound, you should ask a cardiographer to do it for you. That said, when you are scanning a patient with a pleural effusion (Figure 5.2), you may be alerted to the need to get an echocardiogram if you see a dark rim of fluid around the heart.

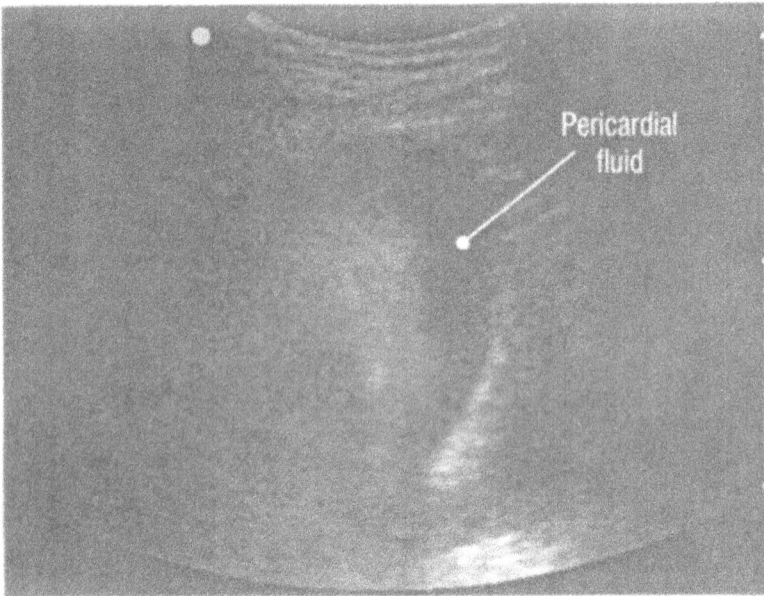

Figure 5.2 Pericardial effusion

6

Pulmonary embolism

Another common cause of pleural fluid is pulmonary infarction. This is quite difficult to see with ultrasound, but you may occasionally see the characteristic appearance of a triangular lucent area next to the effusion. The black area may have a central white spot.

These appearances are insufficient to make a firm diagnosis of pulmonary embolism, but might prompt you to arrange further imaging.

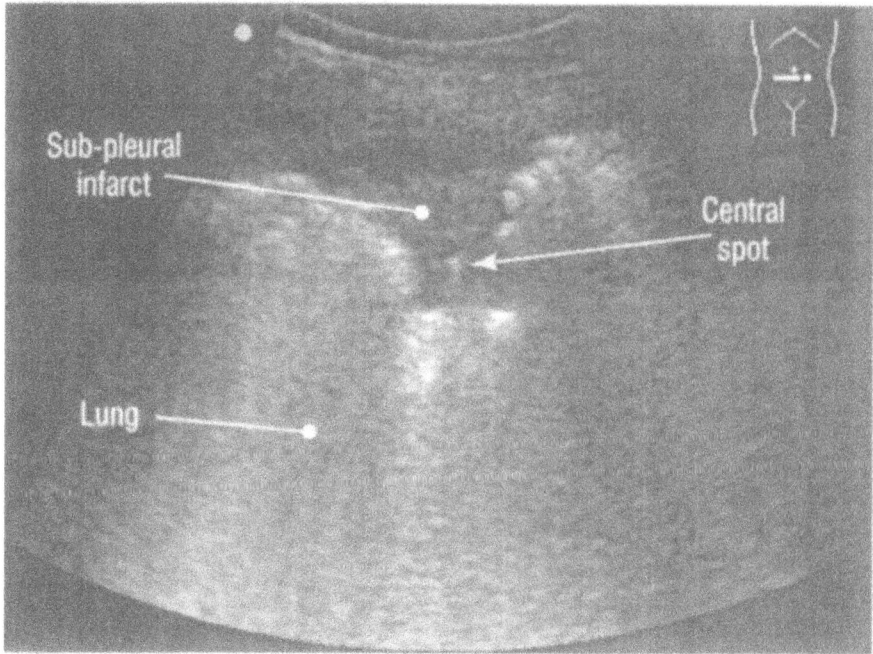

Figure 6.1 Pulmonary infarct.

Flare artefact

Time for another artefact. We have already noted how ultrasound waves pass easily through water. When they encounter underlying lung, this will sometimes appear very bright because there is so much more ultrasound still present, compared to adjacent lung where the ultrasound waves have been attenuated as they pass through the overlying air-filled lung. This is called a flare artefact.

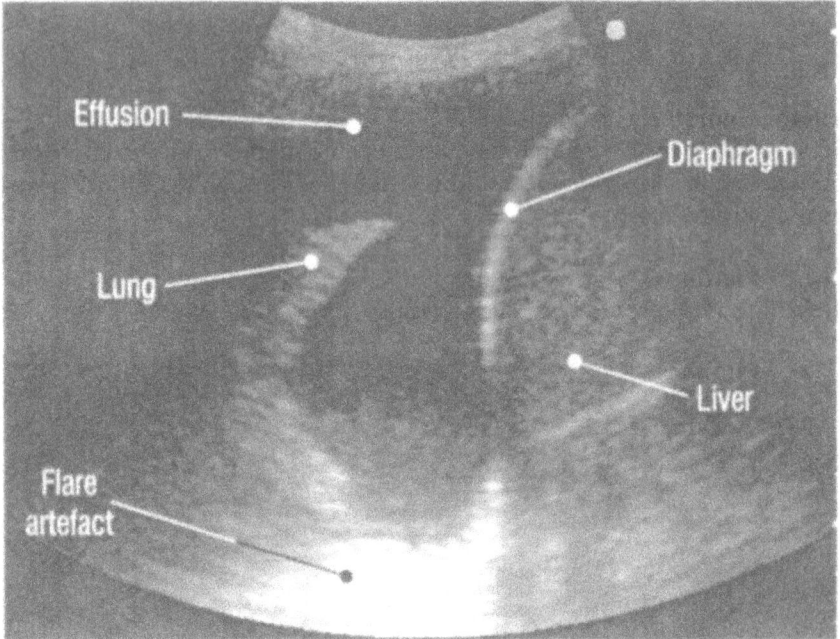

Figure 6.2 Flare artefact.

7

Pleural thickening

For the next sections of this book, we'll be looking at more superficial structures – the pleura, ribs and lymph nodes. The "abdominal" probe we have used up until now is fine for this purpose, but if you have a smaller , higher frequency probe – for example, one normally used for central line placement – then you will probably get better pictures of these more superficial structures.

In order to get used to the new probe, let's go back to looking at the liver. Using the abdominal probe, scan your own liver in the same way as we did in section 2 and set the depth to the most shallow setting.

Now change the probe to the higher frequency one, and see if you get better definition.

Palpate an intercostal space, then hold the probe at a right-angle to the space. You should see the ribs above and below the space: the outer cortex of the rib reflects the ultrasound waves and creates the rib shadows we have noted previously. Between the ribs, you will see the intercostal muscles and pleura.

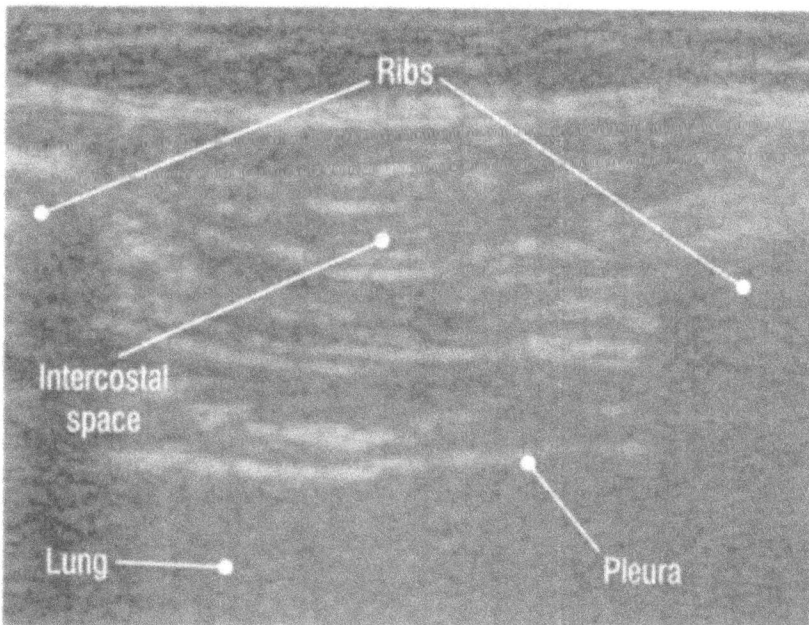

Figure 7.1 Ribs and intercostal space

Slide to and fro over the rib and intercostal space until you are clear about the anatomical appearances.

One key appearance is sliding of the visceral pleural surface with respiration. This is impossible to show you with still images. When you have a clear image of the intercostal space, watch carefully until you are sure you can recognise pleural sliding.

Loss of this normal sliding appearance is a good indicator of significant pleural pathology, for example when a lung tumour is invading through to the chest wall, or in the presence of a pneumothorax.

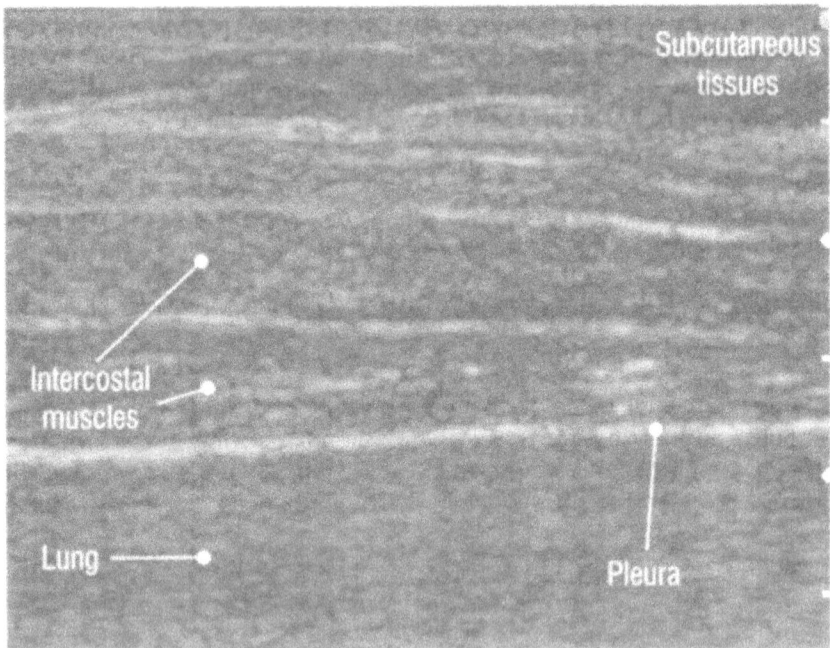

Figure 7.2 Intercostal space.

Perhaps surprisingly, pleural thickening is difficult to detect, particularly in the absence of a pleural effusion, and is only easily apparent when it is more than a centimetre in thickness.

Differentiating benign (Figure 7.3) and malignant (Figure 7.4) pleural thickening is difficult, unless you see erosion into bone or the chest wall– we'll discuss this when we look at the ribs.

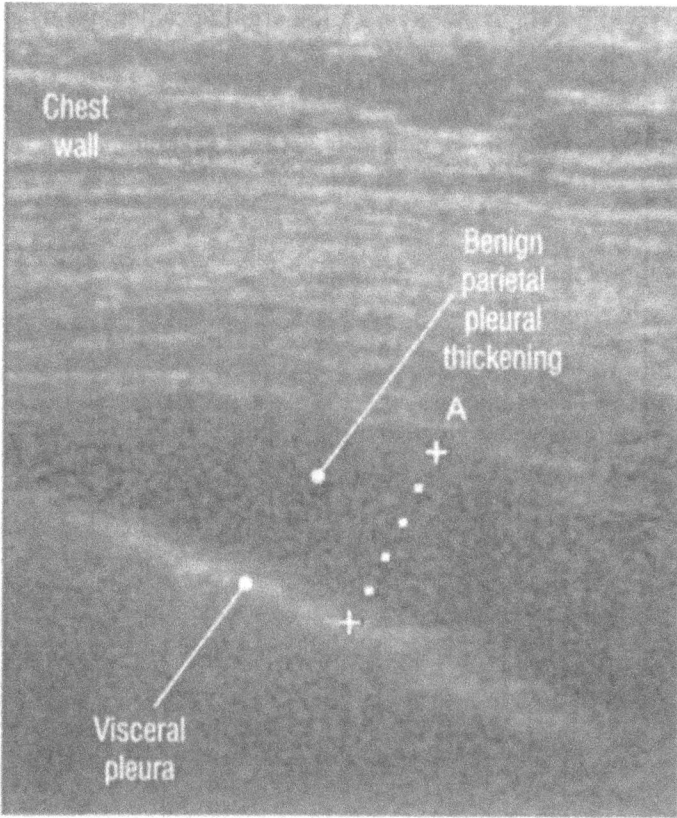

Figure 7.3 Benign pleural thickening.

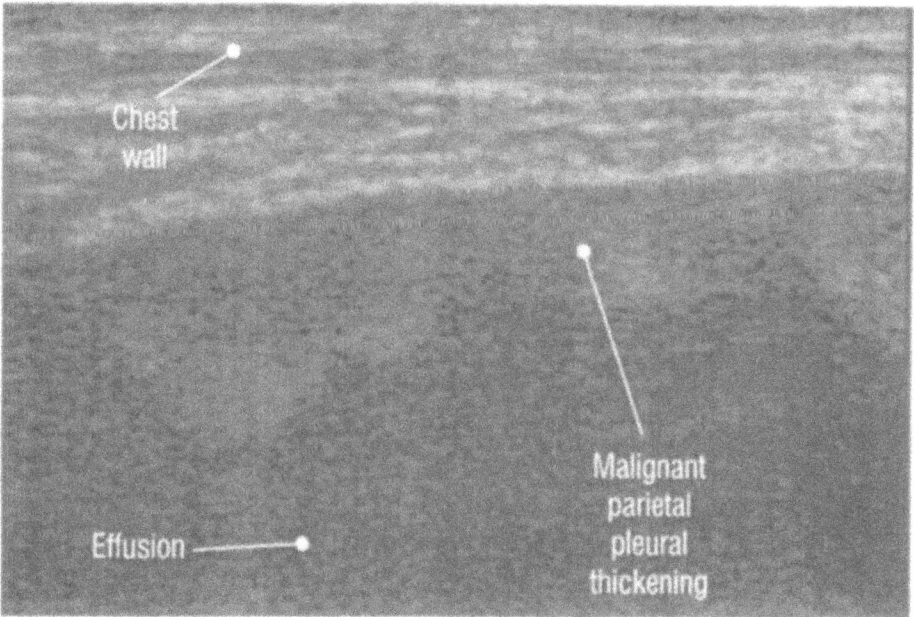

Figure 7.4 Malignant pleural thickening.

A few pointers to a benign aetiology for pleural thickening are as follows:

- Uniformly dark (ie non-echogenic) appearance
- Smooth edge
- White flecks of calcium within black pleural thickening
- Less than 1cm in thickness

Malignant pleural thickening is more likely with:

- Greater than 1cm in thickness
- Irregular margin
- Non-uniform echogenicity
- Loss of sliding between visceral and parietal pleura

8

Pneumothorax

Ultrasound is good for looking at things that contain water. Air blocks the conduction of ultrasound, so you cannot see a pneumothorax with ultrasound.

When you have a lot of experience in ultrasounding the chest, you may be able to infer the presence of a pneumothorax, but this is much more difficult than anything we've done so far.

Start by scanning patients you know have a large pneumothorax, in the same way as we started with large pleural effusions. When you are confident that you can identify a pneumothorax, you could begin to use ultrasound in situations where you cannot immediately get a CXR. This may be the case in the emergency department, for example in a patient in whom you suspect a tension pneumothorax if there is no time to get a chest X-ray. Another use is in the intensive care unit, when a ventilated patient suddenly deteriorates and you want to check if they have developed a pneumothorax.

In the presence of a pneumothorax, you do not see the superficial parietal pleura gliding over the visceral pleura, and the underlying echoes tend not to move with respiration – this appearance is sometimes called "frozen echoes". These appearances are impossible to demonstrate in a book with single images.

Other clues to the presence of a pneumothorax are reverberation lines and the disappearance of comet-tail lines. You may well have noticed some white lines on your scans, and now is probably a good time to work out what these are.

Reverberations

Reverberation lines are curved transverse lines seen across the screen, the distance between the lines being equal.

The explanation for these artefacts is quite simple. The ultrasound waves bounce off the pleura back to the probe; the probe "sees" this – correctly - as the pleural surface. Some of the returning ultrasound waves bounce off the probe back to the pleura – and back again; because they have made the journey to the pleura and back twice, it takes twice as long for them to get back to the probe.

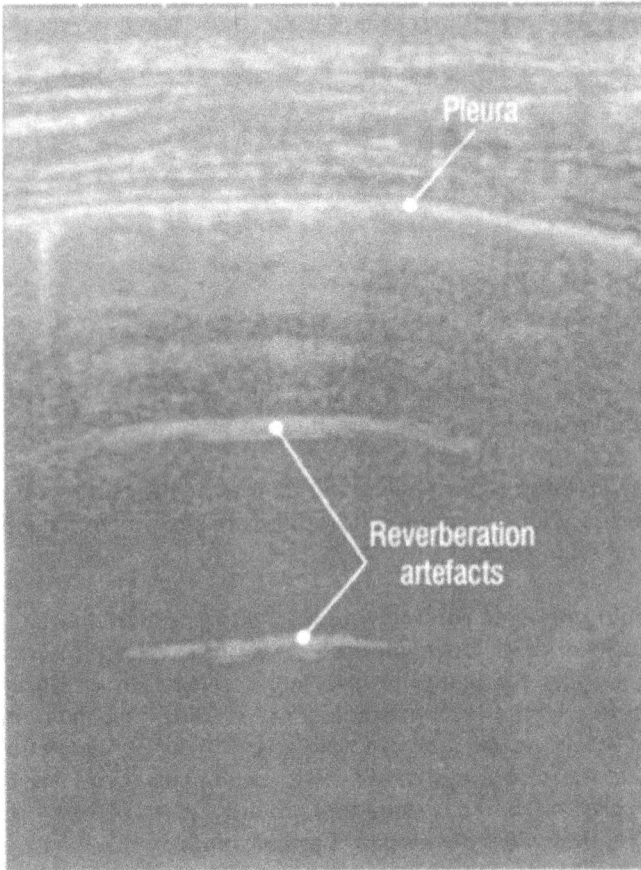

Figure 8.1 Reverberation lines. The two deeper lines are not real structures, but artefacts created by resonance.

The probe interprets this – incorrectly – as a second reflector twice as far away as the pleura. If the ultrasound waves bounce three times, the probe "sees" a third reflector three times as deep.

You may see reverberation artefacts in other situations, for example in Figure 12.1 there are several false images of the aspiration needle.

Reverberation between two thickened interlobular septa may well be the explanation for the comet-tail artefacts we saw in Figure 5.1.

Rib fractures can also generate reverberation artefacts.

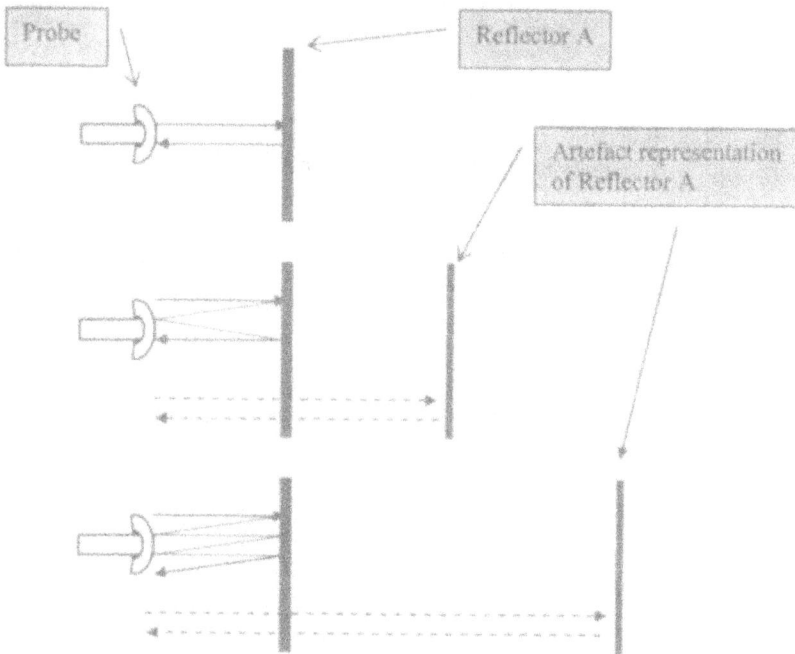

Figure 8.2 The physical explanation of reverberation artefacts.

Surgical emphysema

Subcutaneous air pockets reflect ultrasound waves, so in the presence of surgical emphysema you will see nothing in the deeper tissues.

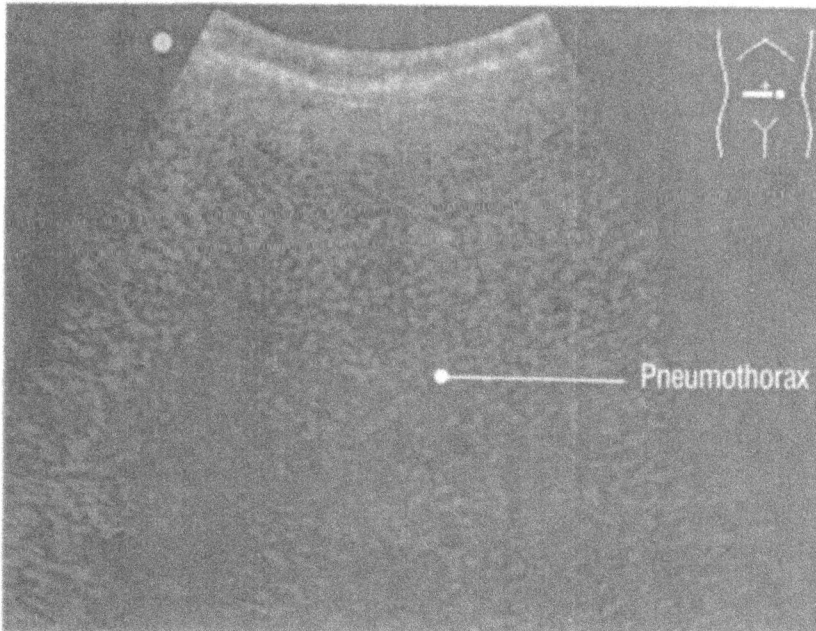

Figure 8.3 Subcutaneous emphysema. The screen will appear "frozen", with no movement during respiration.

This appearance is sometimes called a "frozen" screen: there is nothing much to see, and there is no movement of the echoes when the patient breathes in and out.

You may be asked to scan the chest of a patient with a chest drain in place, to see if all the pleural fluid has been removed. This is seldom helpful because there is usually some air in the pleural space, which blocks your view.

As with pleural effusions, it is probably best to start with a patient you already know to have a large pneumothorax. Scan both sides of the chest anteriorly, starting at the top in the mid-clavicular line and moving down over the lungs. Hopefully you will be able to see the differences between the two sides.

Picking up a small pneumothorax in a patient with COPD can be difficult, if there is a lot of air trapped in the lungs at the apices, with little pleural movement.

9

Ribs

We noted right at the start that the ribs block ultrasound waves, leaving shadows behind them.

With the probe parallel to the ribs, slide the probe over rib and intercostal space alternately until you can recognise the bright reflections from the outer cortex of the rib.

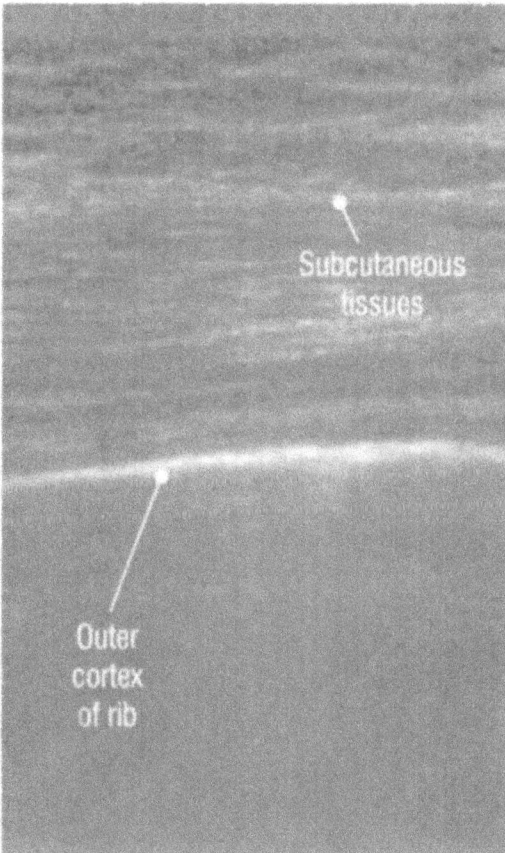

Figure 9.1 Outer cortex of normal rib.

If there is a fracture, you may see a step in the cortex of the bone. You may see this if you scan carefully over an area where the patient is experiencing pain.

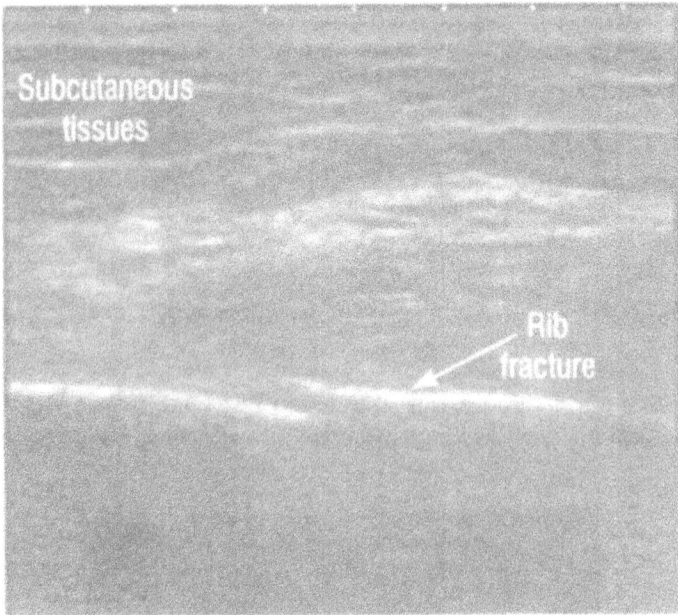

Figure 9.2 Fractured rib.

If the bone of the rib is destroyed – for example, by tumour – it will be possible to see through the rib.

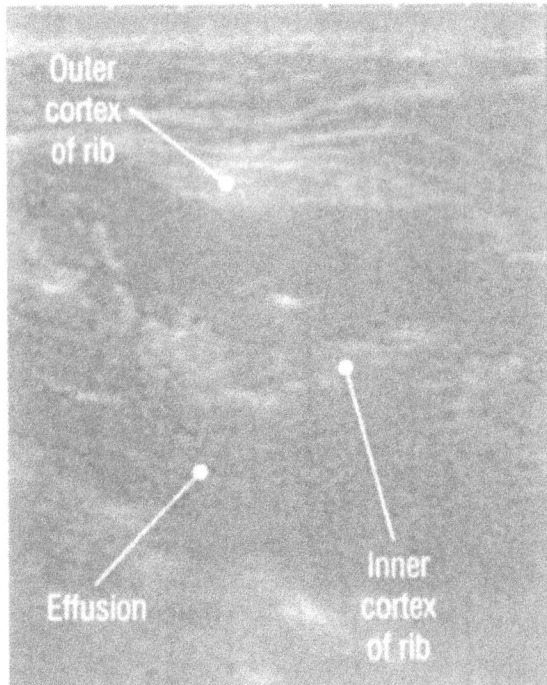

Figure 9.3 Rib metastasis.

A word of caution about costo-chondral junctions: the change from bone to cartilage may mimic bone erosion, with the rib becoming lucent. Sometimes you can see calcification within the cartilage.

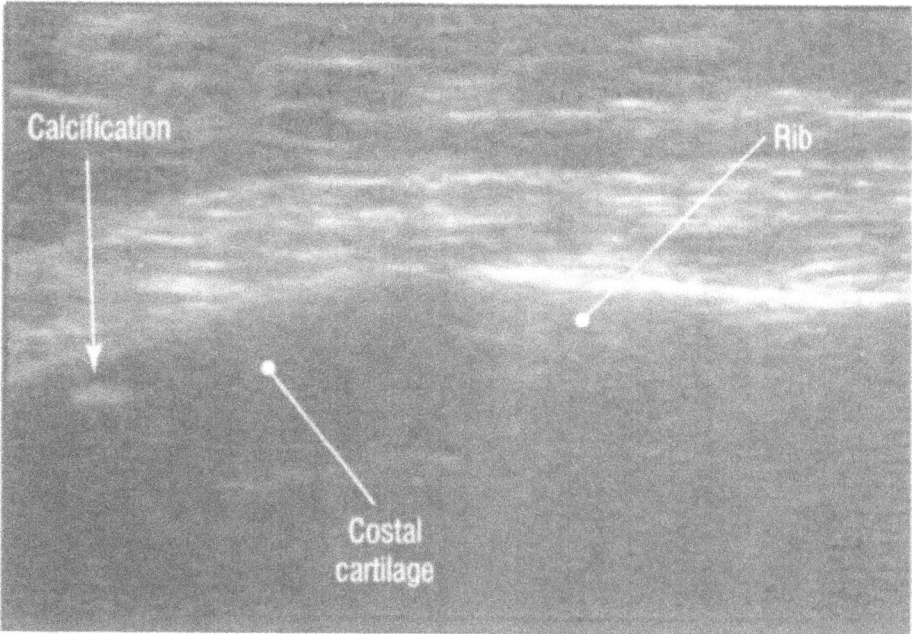

Figure 9.4 Costo-chondral junction.

10
Lymph Nodes

You may already be able to perform needle aspiration of enlarged cervical lymph nodes. You don't need ultrasound if they are palpable, although sometimes a scan will show their exact location and morphology.

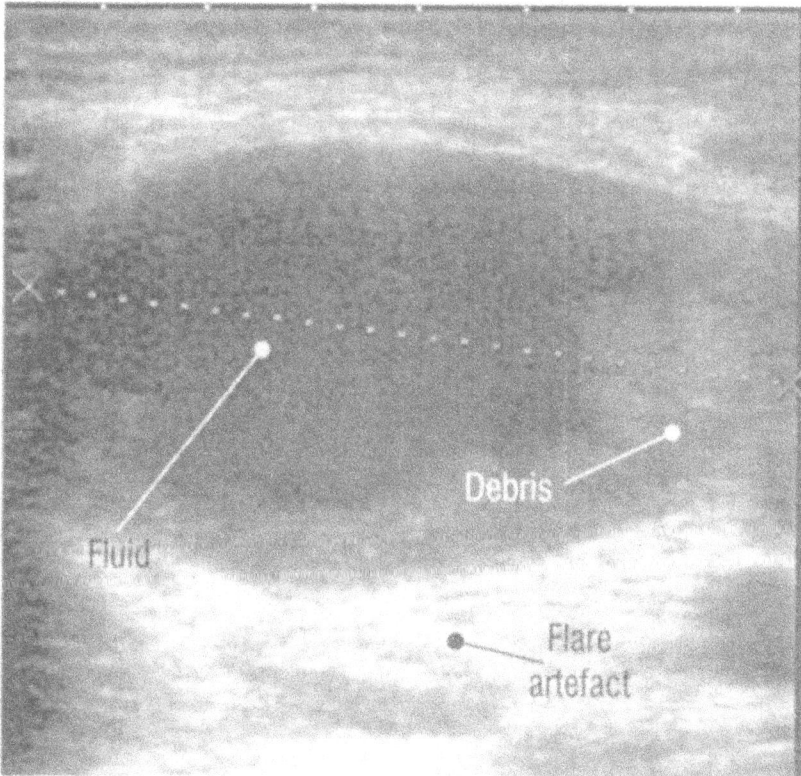

Figure 10.1 Pus within a tuberculous cervical lymph node, or "cold abscess".

Scanning a palpable node may help you tell whether it is malignant. A non-malignant lymph node is oval, smooth, with a central echo from hilar fat.

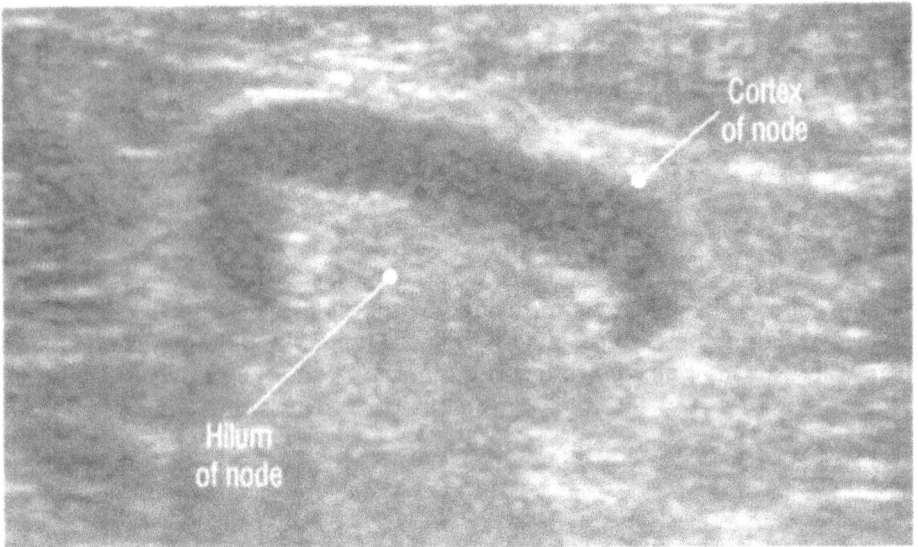

Figure 10.2 Non-malignant lymph node.

A malignant node is more round, less regular, and the hilar echo is lost.

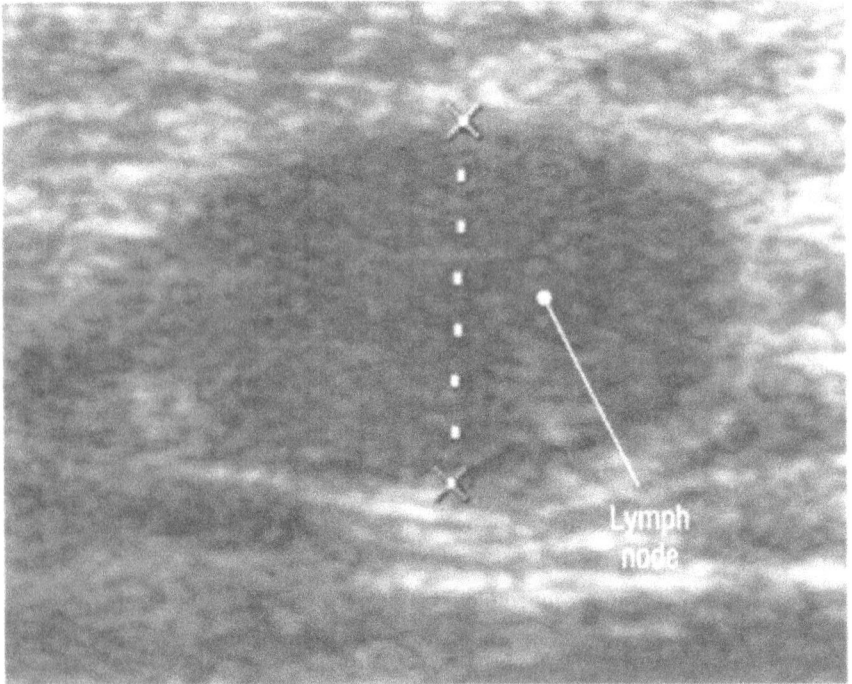

Figure 10.3 Malignant lymph node.

Pathological nodes may have a dark rim around them, indicating oedema or "periadenitis".

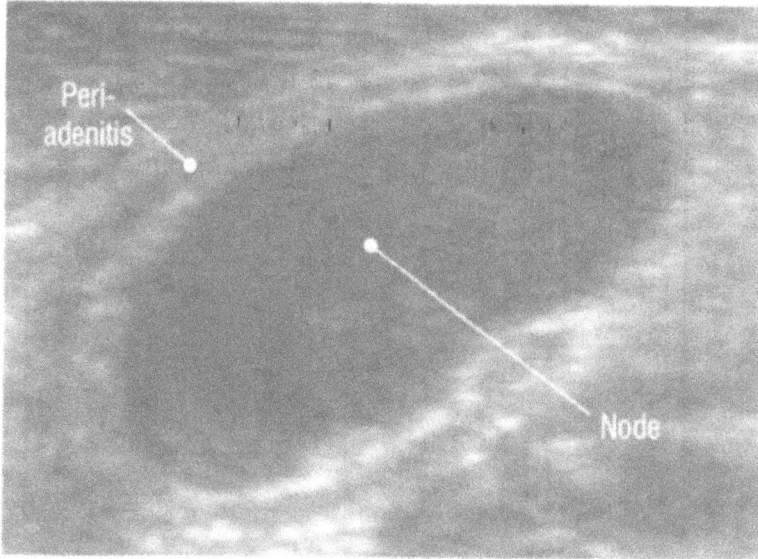

Figure 10.4 Oedema around a pathological lymph node.

With ultrasound, you will pick up smaller non-palpable nodes which may be amenable to biopsy.

When you are scanning pleural effusions you may see pathological nodes in the adjacent chest wall, which may indicate a malignant process.

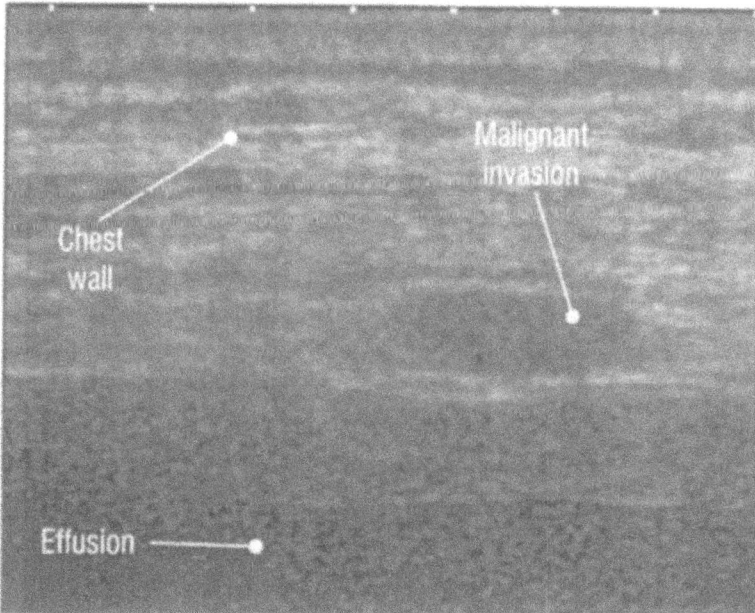

Figure 10.5 Extra-pleural lymph node.

Doppler ultrasound can be used to detect an abnormal blood flow within a lymph node. Benign nodes have flow only at the hilum, whereas a malignant node has peripheral flow aswell.

11

The Diaphragm

Finding the diaphragm is a central part of orientating yourself when you are scanning the chest, so by now you will be quite familiar with what a normal diaphragm looks like.

If the diaphragm looks irregular and thickened (particularly if it is >7mm) then the likelihood of malignancy increases.

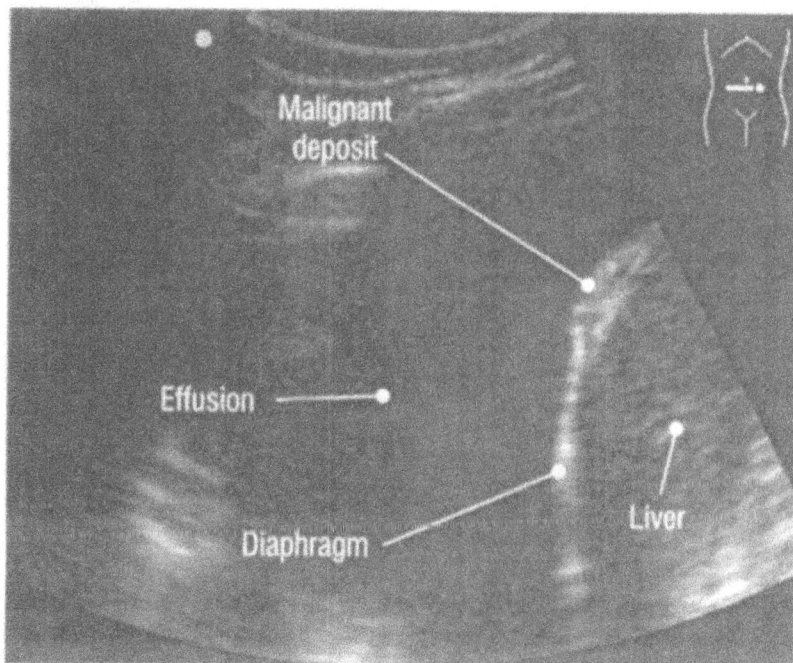

Figure 11.1 Malignant infiltration of the diaphragm.

Ultrasound can be used to look at the movement of the diaphragm. During inspiration, the diaphragm descends and thickens.

You can ask the patient to sniff – if the diaphragm is paralysed, it should move upwards when the pressure inside the chest is negative. This is called paradoxical motion: normally the diaphragm descends when you sniff, because of active contraction of the muscle, but when it is paralysed it just flops upwards because of the negative pressure created inside the chest by the remaining inspiratory muscles. In practice, this is not a very sensitive way of picking up diaphragm paralysis.

In the presence of diaphragmatic herniation, bowel can be seen in the chest. This is much easier to see in real-time, when there is peristalsis of the bowel.

Mirror-image artefacts

Time for one last artefact. The diaphragm is a strong reflector, which leads to the "mirror" artefact, whereby you see a structure on both sides of the diaphragm, one of the images being a mirror-image.

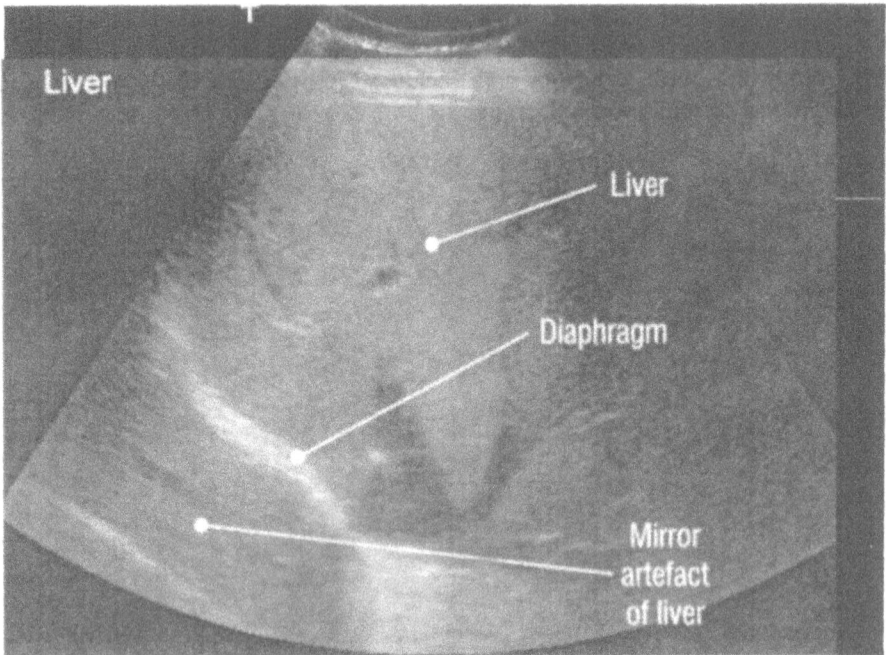

Figure 11.2 Mirror-image artefact of liver

The first, true image of the liver is represented correctly. The second, false image is caused by reflection off the diaphragm: the ultrasound waves take longer to travel along this longer path, so the probe "sees" the second image as being deeper, beyond the diaphragm.

If you look carefully, you will see faint mirror artefacts quite commonly whenever there is a strongly reflective surface.

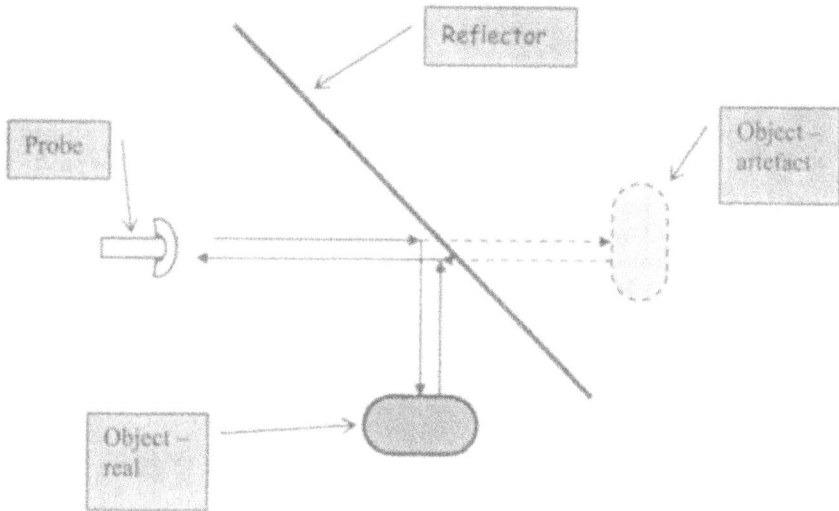

Figure 11.3 Physics of mirror artefact

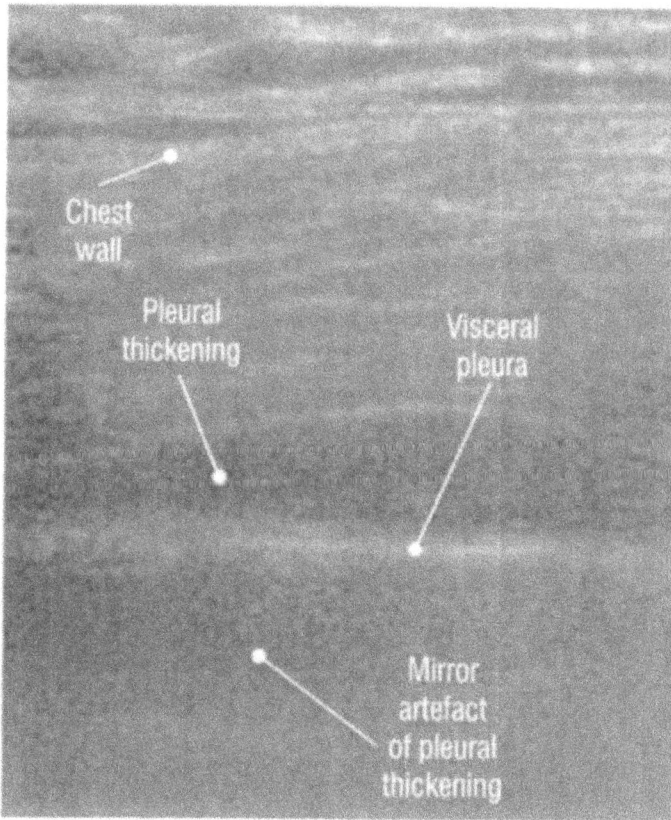

Figure 11.4 Mirror artefact of pleural thickening.

12

Interventional Ultrasound

Pleural aspiration

We have already seen how to use ultrasound to identify the site for a pleural aspiration or chest drain insertion, performing the procedure conventionally after the scan. By placing a sterile plastic sheath over the ultrasound probe, it is possible to aspirate under direct ultrasound guidance. This is useful when a pleural effusion is very small or loculated (in which case aspirate the largest or deepest pocket of fluid).

Insert the needle in the same plane as the probe, and guide the tip into the correct place. Some needles have tips coated in a special polymer which makes them more echogenic ; if you cannot see the tip clearly, move the needle gently from side-to-side. When using the Seldinger technique to insert a pleural drain, the guide wire should be easy to see on ultrasound.

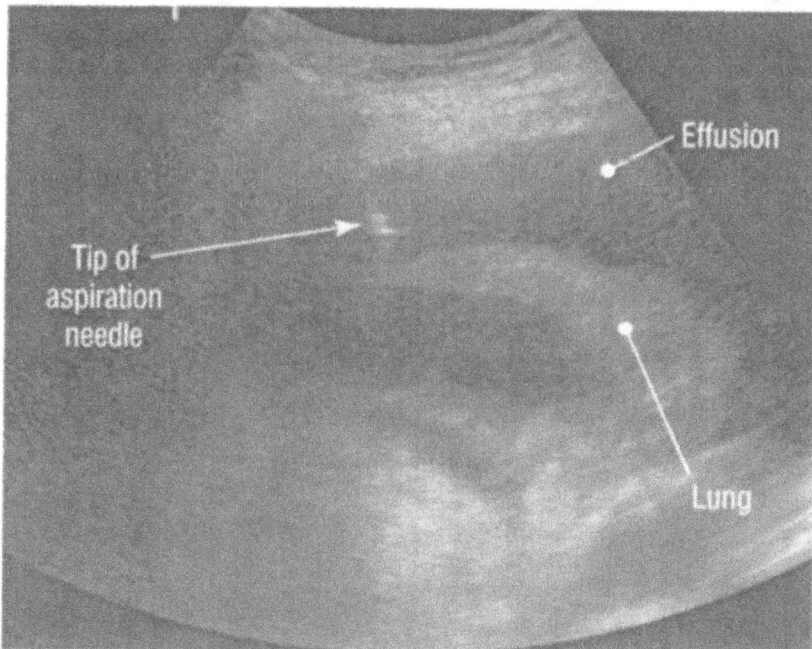

Figure 12.1 Tip of needle in pleural fluid.

Ultrasound-guided biopsy

Ultrasound can be used for biopsy of lymph nodes, rib lesion, pleura and peripheral lung lesions. The approach is similar to that used for pleural aspiration. For pleural and lung lesions, the site and depth for biopsy are checked with the patient breathing quietly; infiltration of local anaesthesia and insertion of the biopsy needle are performed after asking the patient to hold their breath (without a prior deep inspiration, which alters the position of the lesion relative to the skin).

Ultrasound-guided biopsy of supra-clavicular or axillary lymph nodes is a useful technique for obtaining a tissue diagnosis in patients with lung cancer, even if there are no palpable lymph nodes. Colour Doppler can be used to delineate adjacent vascular structures.

Loss of the sliding pleura sign after the procedure can be used to see if a pneumothorax has developed. After the procedure, document in the clinical notes exactly what you did. If an intercostal drain was inserted, give details of how it was secured in place, and – in the case of a locking "pig-tail" catheter-whether it needs to be unlocked when the drain is removed.

If you think the patient requires observations or a chest X-ray after the procedure, give details of the timing of these and the action to be taken.

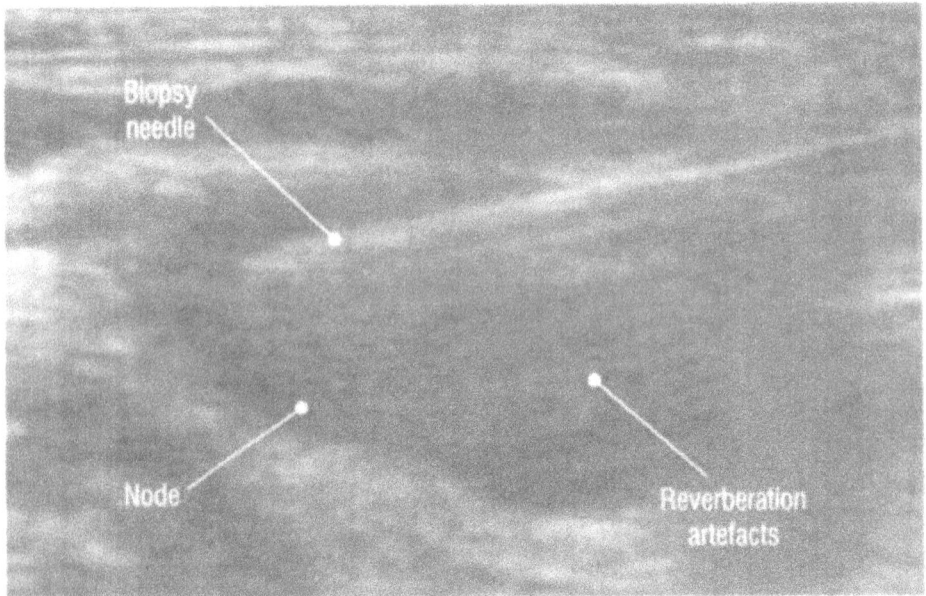

Figure 12.2 Tip of needle in lymph node.

Endnote

Once you start scanning the chest using ultrasound, you will probably never want to aspirate fluid or drain a pleural effusion "blind" ever again. It is a great tool, which will enhance your clinical practice. Use it wisely.

In order to become competent, you need some theoretical background, which we hope this book provides. You also need to do lots of scans. Initially you will need supervision. Even when you have done lots of scans, there will be appearances which puzzle you. If you can, save an image and show it to an expert. Even better, get them to scan the patient and show you what they see.

Know your limitations. Unless you are a radiologist, you will mainly be looking at pleural effusions. You may see the heart, kidneys, liver or lots of other structures when you scan the chest, but don't be tempted to stray into interpreting what you see unless you have been specifically trained to do so. Of course if you see what you think might be a pericardial effusion or liver abscess, you should get an expert to scan the relevant area.

Further Reading

Agricola E, Bove T, Oppizzi M, Marino G, Zangrillo A, Margonato A, Picano E. "Ultrasound comet-tail images": a marker of pulmonary edema. *Chest* 2005;127:1690-1695.

Beckh S, Bolcskei P, Lessnau K-D. Real-time chest ultrasonography. A comprehensive review for the pulmonologist. *Chest* 2002;122:1759-1773.

Chen KY, Liaw YS, Wang HC, et al. Sonographic septation: a useful prognostic indicator of acute thoracic empyema. *J Ultrasound Med* 2000;19:837-843.

Chian CF, Su WL, Soh LH et al. Echogenic swirling pattern as a predictor of malignant pleural effusions in patients with malignancies. *Chest* 2004;126:129-134.

Feller-Kopman D. Pleural ultrasound. *Thorax* 2009;64:97-98.

Feller-Kopman D. Ultrasound-guided thoracentesis. *Chest* 2006;129:1709-1714.

Gorg C, Restrepo I, Schwerk WB. Sonography of malignant pleural effusion. *Eur J Radiol* 1997;7:1195-1198.

Grogan DR, Irwin RS, Channick R, et al. Complications associated with thoracentesis. A prospective, randomized study comparing three different methods. *Arch Intern Med* 1990;150:873-877.

Hirsch JH, Rogers JV, Mack LA. Real-time sonography of pleural opacities. *Am J Roentgenol* 1981;136:297-301.

Light RW. *Pleural Diseases*, 5th edition. Lippincott, Williams and Wilkins, Phildadelphia 2007. ISBN 978-0-7817-6957-0

Jaffe A, Calder AD, Owens CM, Stanojevic, S, Sonnappa S. Role of routine computed tomography in paediatric pleural empyema. *Thorax* 2008;63:897-902.

Kumaran M, Benamore RE, Vaidhyanath R, Muller S, Richards CJ, Peake MD, Entwisle JJ. Ultrasound guided cytological aspiration of supraclavicular lymph nodes in patients with suspected lung cancer. *Thorax* 2005;60:229-33.

Mathis G. *Chest Sonography*. Springer, New York 2007. ISBN 978-3540724-27-8.

Mayo PH, Doelken P. Pleural ultrasonography. *Clin Chest Med* 2206; 27: 215-227.

Mayo PH. Goltz HR, Tafreshi M et al. Safety of ultrasound-guided thoracentesis in patients receiving mechanical ventilation. *Chest* 2004;125:1059-1062.

Quereshi NR, Gleeson FV. Imaging of pleural disease. *Clin Chest Med* 2006;27:193-213.

Quereshi NR, Rahman NM, Gleeson FV. Thoracic ultrasound in the diagnosis of malignant pleural effusion. *Thorax* 2009;64:139-143.

Ultrasound training recommendations for medical and surgical specialities. Royal College of Radiologists, London 2004. www.rcr.ac.uk

Yabng PC, Luh KT, Chang DB et al. Value of sonography in determining the nature of pleural effusion: analysis of 320 cases. *Am J Roentgenol* 1992;159:29-33.

Index